Breast Beating

A personal odyssey in the quest for an understanding of breast cancer, the meaning of life and other easy questions

By

Michael Baum MB, FRCS, ChM, MD, FRCR
Professor emeritus of surgery

And

Visiting professor of medical humanities
University College London
michael@mbaum.freeserve.co.uk

Dedicated to the memory of
Professor David Baum FRCP, MD, PRCPCH
1940–1999
My Best Man

Acknowledgements

I wish firstly to acknowledge the devoted loyalty of my wife Judy through the thick and thin of my turbulent career. In addition, to thank her for proof reading and giving wise advice on the contents of my story. Next I wish to acknowledge the inspiration for my long journey provided by my devoted mother Mary, who denied herself so much in order to care for and bring up a large family during the tough times of the Second World War and its aftermath of austerity, only to die in uncontrolled pain from advanced breast cancer at the early age of 67. My loving sister Linda, who fortunately has fared better than our mother with the challenge of breast cancer, is the perfect exemplar of the courage of thousands of women worldwide suffering from this disease. She and others like her have been my continuing source of inspiration. I thank my brothers Geoffrey and Harold for being such wonderful role models, my children Richard, Katie and Suzanne for making me so proud, and my grandchildren, Ellie, Josh, Rafi, Zack, Sam, Theo, Leo, Joe and Jake (in descending order of age, I think) for making me smile whenever the going got tough.

I also must thank my publishers, Andrew and Shan White, for placing their trust in me and for their brilliant editorial work.

Finally I must thank the thousands of women with breast cancer who selflessly offered themselves up for clinical trials for the sake of future generations, without them no progress would have been made and without whom my career would have foundered.

Published in the UK by:

Anshan Ltd
11a Little Mount Sion
Tunbridge Wells
Kent. TN1 1YS

Tel: +44 (0) 1892 557767
Fax: +44 (0) 1892 530358

e-mail: info@anshan.co.uk
web site: www.anshan.co.uk

ISBN: 978 1 848290 42 6

British Library Cataloguing in Publication Data
A catalogue record for this book is available from the British Library.

Copy Editor: Andrew White
Cover Design: Terry Griffiths
Typeset by: GCS, Leighton Buzzard, Bedfordshire

Contents

List of figures

Foreword

by Nick Ross

Breasts are the most visibly defining characteristics of a woman, and cancer is one of the most chilling diagnoses in medicine. The combination makes for an emotive brew. Michael Baum has spent his professional career trying to tease out the facts about breast cancer from the swirl of medical and sexual politics. What causes it? How does it spread? And, above all, how can we best conquer it? Prof Baum brings to the quest a precious combination of passion and intellectual detachment. His research has caused him to question many of the things he was taught at medical school and that he learned as a junior doctor from master surgeons and physicians. It has caused him to change his own mind and even, very publicly, to reverse his line on policies that he once championed. It has led him to battle orthodoxies in conventional medicine and to revile claims made for complementary and alternative therapies.

I first encountered Michael Baum some twenty years ago when I agreed, with some reluctance, to spend three days trying to adjudicate an argument among doctors. Breast cancer was one of the most pernicious killers of women, and any consensus on how to treat it had broken down. So Britain's leading healthcare think-tank invited the quarrelsome experts to assemble in London and make their case to a medical jury. The panel consisted mostly of surgeons and physicians, all noted in their field but none involved directly with treating breast cancer. I was one of the lay members.

Those three days turned out to be one of the most eye-opening experiences of my life.

We all like to think that doctors know what they're doing, and that what they're doing is firmly based in medical science. But the experts who appeared before us, all confident and all firm in their convictions (and all men as I recall), seemed mostly to rely on anecdote, on what they had learned as students, and on personal experience. Where are the data, we asked? Where is the evidence that your approach is superior at saving lives or mitigating the worst effects of cancer? Again and again we were told that we should trust their judgement. Some of the experts championed super-radical mastectomies, a mutilating procedure that removes the breast, the lymph nodes in the armpit, and a good deal more besides, and so can result in the patient being disabled as well as disfigured. Anything less, they warned, would leave cancer cells in the patient, which was tantamount to killing them. Other surgeons advocated rather less injurious procedures and some proposed simply taking out the lump. Radiologists suggested radiotherapy, physicians wanted chemotherapy. Everyone was polite, but plainly passions ran high, as well they might. Lives were at stake, and so were reputations and deeply-held beliefs.

Michael Baum was then, and remains, a refreshing voice of reason and compassion. His knowledge of breast cancer is second to none, his willingness to abandon old nostrums in the face of new research is commendable, and his determination – almost enthusiasm – to reject his own ideas when new facts point to new ones is sign of real scientific greatness. Unlike in politics where U-turns are disparaged, in medicine following the evidence is the essence of good patient care. This is a man who believed, as did all mainstream oncologists, that cancer spreads through the lymphatic system. Yet he has been in the vanguard of those who now suspect it spreads through blood. The difference is by no means arcane; it calls for a fundamental reassessment of cancer treatment.

Prof Baum is brave. He has long warned about "the flight from rational thinking" posed by the recycled fashion for alternative medicine lobby. But he is also prepared to take on his own colleagues. He was one of the first to champion cancer screening and then, as inconvenient data emerged, he became one of its most vocal critics, much to the annoyance of many fellow doctors and of the powerful screening lobby groups he himself had helped to create.

This book, as he puts it himself, is really about, "how false assumptions about the nature of breast cancer gave rise to cruel and futile interventions that added to the sum of human suffering."

But, above all, it is a book about human nobility and hope.

Mostly about Mum

The first time I guessed that something was wrong with my mother was when I noticed her clasping her lower back in pain whilst climbing upstairs in front of me. This was in about 1972 on one of my rare visits home during my period of living in Cardiff and the image is burnt in my memory as a result of what was to follow. My mother was extremely stoical and never complained about ill health. Following on my enquiry, she claimed that it was her "rheumatism" playing up. I thought no more about it until about three months later when she was admitted to hospital to have her gall bladder removed because of stones and increasing pains in the region just below the ribs on the right. This was in no way alarming or for that matter surprising, as she fitted the stereotype. She was female, overweight and over forty. In addition she was constantly munching "Rennies" for heartburn, presumably due to reflux oesophagitis (a condition I inherited with a vengeance),that tends to co-exist with gallstones. The operation went all right and she did indeed have gall stones; however in the post operative phase she developed agonizing pain spreading round from her mid lumbar region to the upper abdomen. X rays of her spine showed a crush fracture of the first lumbar vertebra and suspicion of skeletal secondaries from an unsuspected cancer. A rapid and more thorough clinical examination revealed an advanced cancer in her right breast. She was told not to worry as this was only "chronic mastitis" but my father was contacted immediately and told the grim news. My dad then contacted his five children, three of whom were medically qualified, to pass on the news, and begged us not to let on to mum that she had cancer that had spread round the body. To my lasting shame I concurred with this charade. Opiates were the only way of controlling her pain in the short term although radiotherapy to the spine provided more lasting benefit. The chemotherapy was harsh, causing nausea, vomiting, fatigue and the permanent loss of her long glossy black hair. I was not aware of any benefit from this cruel cocktail. After about twelve months the pains started up again and became more and more difficult to control. It reached the point when, according to erroneous belief at the time, (that adequate analgesia would suppress her breathing and accelerate her demise), escalating doses of opiates were denied her. At this point the family gathered in London and my opinion was sought. I couldn't bear the sight of her in pain and yet the Jewish teaching was clear on this point; as life is of infinite worth and as you cannot split infinity, then every moment of life was of equal value. She therefore continued to suffer until neither she nor the family could take any more and she died within 6 hours of a dose of morphine that adequately controlled her pain. She died on my 37th birthday, May 31st 1974.

The Jewish tradition has it that the dead must be buried within 24 hours and until then the body must not be left alone. I spent the nightlong vigil with my father and had plenty of time to confront my conscience, firstly for not having done enough to help her and secondly for not having demonstrating a son's love at the time she needed it most.

Every mother loves her sons unconditionally but the return of such love by a son is often conditional and context dependent. At the time of my mother's terminal illness I was very self absorbed. My duties as a senior lecturer/consultant surgeon at the University Hospital of Wales were onerous and occupied me for about ten hours a day not counting a one in three rota for night time emergencies. I was very ambitious, setting up research programmes, raising grants and keeping my eyes open for the chance of a professorial appointment. I often worked all weekends keeping up to date with the medical journals, writing manuscripts and dealing with correspondence. What little time I had left was lavished on my wife and three children under 7. I had no more space for love beyond this narrow circle and resented the distraction of my mother's illness at the time. I loved her as a dependent child, was embarrassed by her hats on parent's day when I was a school boy, had little time for her as a young professional but came to admire and yes, love her most of all, in retrospect, since her death. (Figure 1)

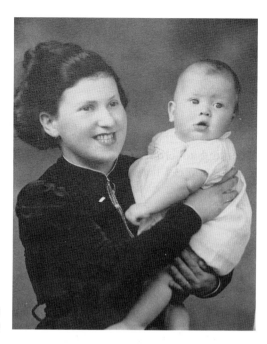

Fig. 1 Me as baby in mother's arms

My mother was a true *ayshet chayil*[1], who dedicated her whole life to the family, the most selfless person I have ever known. During the dark days of the war, the blitz and rationing, she looked after four children of her own (my sister was born after the war) together with other orphans, waifs and strays. From negligible resources she conjured up spectacular *haimishe* (Yiddish homely) meals, made her own cream cheese, *lokshen* (noodles) and *kichelers* (biscuits) from basic raw materials. In the absence of any household appliances she boiled all the linen in a great bubbling cauldron of a tub, extracted the last mote of dirt from the wet clothing and bed sheets on a scrubbing board, squeezed out the water in a huge mangle like a primitive printing press and hung it all out to dry either in the roof on a pulley system or if the weather was fine on a line in the yard. The heavy pre-modern irons were heated on the hot surface of the range (a pre-modern kind of Aga) and heaved on to the ironing board that was in constant use. Her obsessive personality (something else I've also inherited with a vengeance) meant that everything had to be folded and filed away in its place before she collapsed into bed after midnight. By the time I rose in the morning, the coal-fuelled range was alight, water had been boiled and a hearty breakfast prepared to keep us insulated from the cold on our walk to school.

She was not a conventionally beautiful woman, but apple cheeks, dimples and an endearing smile radiated warmth and internal loveliness. From her forties onwards she was stout, but in those days even the most fashion conscious women relied on whale bone rather than "weightwatchers" to define their waist and redistribute the fat above and below the belt. She was always smartly "turned out" and would never be seen out of doors without makeup and a feather in her rakish hat. Most of all though she prided herself on her long black hair, which she assured me came down to her waist. I could never confirm this as she was too proud to leave her bedroom without her hair fixed up in a complex chignon secured in place like a Japanese Geisha girl. The loss of her hair, and its replacement with a silk scarf, was the final insult that the cancer could hurl at her; and for what purpose?

One evening, 20 years after my mother's death, I received a phone call from my sister Linda, then aged 48. She explained that she had just noticed a lump in her right breast, her GP had referred her to the local surgeon who had reassured her but arranged for a biopsy in about two months time. By this time I was Professor of surgery at the Royal Marsden Hospital in London, the most prestigious specialist cancer centre in the UK. I swallowed hard and suggested that she got a second opinion from Mr. Nigel Sacks, a man I trusted because as my senior lecturer I had witnessed the care and skill of his practice first hand. It has to be understood that I couldn't examine my own sister or trust my own judgment, in part out of decorum and in part out of emotional involvement. He saw her the next day and completed the "triple assessment"; that is clinical examination, X rays and a needle biopsy. Within the hour her cancer was diagnosed! Within the week she had surgery that consisted of a "lumpectomy" and partial excision of the lymph nodes in her right axilla. She was home in two days and happily the pathology was favorable. The margins of excision were clear of disease, the tumour was low grade and hormone receptor positive (see chapter 13) and finally the lymph nodes were declared free of malignant deposits. She was started on tamoxifen which she took without side effects for 5 years and underwent a 6 weeks course of radiotherapy to the breast. Without tempting providence I'm happy to say that 12 years later she is still alive and well and still my lovely sister Linda, who follows in my mother's footsteps as an *ayshet chayil*. She has four vivacious daughters who I adore and I think they reciprocate my love. She also has a vivacious dog with which I share a relationship of mutual distaste.

Without wishing to over-dramatize the case, I feel that to some extent I've expunged a little of the guilt I felt over my failure to help my mother. I transferred my sister's care to a top specialist and expedited her diagnosis and treatment. Most of all I have to take some satisfaction in having lead the team that first demonstrated that the drug tamoxifen could reduce breast cancer mortality. (see chapter 8).

Two years ago Linda's oldest daughter came to see me for advice. I'm sure she wouldn't mind me describing her as theatrical in all senses of the word, but on this occasion I felt that her anxieties were legitimate. Her mother and grandmother had breast cancer and the circumstances of her great grandmother's death also gave rise to concern. In addition we are of *Ashkenazi* extraction. All this hinted at the possibility of a germ line mutation in the BRCA gene pool which if present could lead to an 80% lifetime chance of developing breast cancer (see chapter 14). I referred her on to my friend Ros Eeles, a leading cancer geneticist at the Royal Marsden Hospital, who agreed that the family pedigree did suggest a risk of carrying a breast cancer predisposition gene. With counseling and agreement from the whole family my sister was tested for the *"Ashkenazi"* mutations on BRCA 1 and BRCA 2 (see chapter 14). To everyone's relief Linda was not found to be a carrier.

This story of three generations of my family neatly encapsulates the evolving story of progress in the fight against breast cancer over the forty years since I got involved in the campaign. My mother was too ignorant and/or modest to be aware of the disease. Cancer the "big C" was not talked about or considered almost a stigma close to that associated with "a spot on the lung", the euphemism for tuberculosis. Euphemisms for breast cancer were legion including chronic mastitis, neoplasia, mitotic lesions and at worst a "tumour", that literally means nothing more than a swelling. As a result of all this most cancers presented in a late stage either already inoperable or with overt distant spread (metastases). Even if operable the surgery would be a mutilating Halsted radical mastectomy (see chapter 6). With no malice intended, women were considered too emotionally fragile to handle the truth, so the diagnosis and treatment were discussed with the husband and sons. (I still encounter this cultural mindset with some of my private patients from Pakistan, Saudi Arabia and the Gulf states). Finally palliative care and symptom control were poorly developed and patients suffered unnecessarily. The myth that adequate opiate analgesia shortens life has now been exploded; in fact the opposite is true. Too little and too late has been replaced by adequate and in good time.

By the time my sister presented breast cancer the subject was no longer stigmatized and breast cancer awareness campaigns were making their mark. Diagnosis was available in a "one stop shop" within the hour, matching "Kwikfit" car exhaust replacement for efficiency.

Surgery in most cases can now provide breast conservation with a decent cosmetic outcome without compromising the chance of cure and adjuvant systemic therapy can prolong life or even provide a cure. The development of clinical nurse specialists and the subject of psychosocial-oncology (see chapter 9) have enhanced quality of life, and the developments in palliative care and the hospice movement have improved the "quality of dying".

The experience with my niece provides a pointer to the future. The genetic code for the rare familial predisposition to breast cancer has been cracked. The mechanism that explains why a faulty gene can lead to cancer is understood (see chapter 14) and opportunities for prevention are opening up (see chapter 9). Within a few years I expect the genetic explanation for sporadic breast cancers will be understood and along with that smart ways of preventing the disease will be discovered. In the immediate future we can expect more effective systemic therapy tailored to the individual cancer with specific molecular targets in its aim. Even as I write, tamoxifen the gold standard for thirty years is being replaced by a new class of compound (the aromatase inhibitors) that are not only more effective but carry fewer side effects (see chapter 12).

How all this came about is a fascinating story that touches on the history of medicine, the philosophy of science and the introduction of the humanities into medical education.

This book is also about my life, how it was shaped by the search for an understanding of this enigmatic disease and my modest contributions to the science and treatment of breast cancer. It is also my genuine wish that this story will humanize the subject, demystify the disease, help the afflicted and her family, and most of all offer hope for the future.

Chapter 1

The Importance of Symmetry

Each morning on waking, I get out of bed, turn to my right 90 degrees and find my slippers arranged in perfect symmetry side by side, toes pointing to the mid point of the bed-side table waiting to slide onto my early morning feet. For some reason Judy, my wife, finds this extremely irritating and when making the bed might accidentally on purpose disturb this perfect symmetry with a well placed kick. The curious thing is that I never have any recall of arranging my slippers in this way and yet every morning there they are waiting for me. You may think that's all you need to know about me. Clearly I'm an anal-retentive obsessive neurotic. This was indeed the message contained in a scene of the film "The Dead Poets Society" starring Robin Williams. The protagonist played by Mr. Williams was a free thinking maverick school teacher who ripped pages from textbooks, taught his students to "seize the day" and express their inner self through literature and poetry. The "bad guy" was the father of one of the boys who objected to his son writing poetry and wanting to be an actor when he was destined to join his father's business. He eventually drove his son to suicide and the Robin Williams character was driven out of his job. The "bigoted" father put his slippers on just the way I do and this was shown in close up in order to fix the stereotype. I'm also obsessively tidy in my work practices. My office table is usually cleaned up at the end of each day and any books or papers I'm working from are left beautifully squared off in line with the desktop and arranged in pyramidal piles, largest at the base smallest at the top, looking like a miniature model of the Aztec site outside Mexico City. The desk in my clinic is the same and if I don't see each patient on time I get wound up inside as tight as a watch spring. Like John Cleese in the film "Clockwise", I always try to get there on time. If we have a party to go to that starts at 8.00pm, even if it is the other side of London I always arrive with a chronological precision that even I find uncanny. For some reason my wife finds this habit intensely irritating as well. I must be hard to live with, I'm even hard on myself, yet I can't be all bad as Judy and I have been together for over 40 years and we never row, something else she finds annoying.

Clearly there is an obsessive trait in my character but I would like to say in my defence that part of my love of symmetry is aesthetic in origin. One of my passions in life is fine art, and I paint a bit too. I'm often drawn to paintings in ways I don't at first understand. For example I've just finished a reworking of Vermeer's "Woman Holding a Balance". (Figure 2) I've replaced the pearls that she is weighing with double strands of DNA that also appear in the painting on the wall behind her head in place of the "The Last Judgment", re-naming the painting "The Genetic Test". Only after hours of intense scrutiny

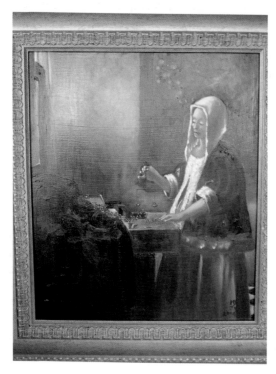

Fig. 2 Copy of Vermeer's painting, Woman holding a balance

did I notice that the fulcrum of the balance that she holds so daintily in her right hand is precisely at the point where the diagonals of the rectangle of the canvas cross. Furthermore if you then follow this point up to the top of the picture and then drop a vertical down to the table top you find you are at the 6 o'clock position of a perfect arc described by a string of pearls looping across the table and the pensive young woman's left arm. That observation gave me as much satisfaction as any scientific discovery.

I'm not quite sure if I was drawn to surgery as a result of this personality trait or whether the years of strict discipline in the operating theatre drove me this way. Certainly many of my colleagues share this behaviour. I love the calm and order in the OR, everything and everyone knowing their place; the instrument tray gleaming with stainless steel reflecting the powerful operating theatre lights, all the instruments lined up in order of size with the consultant surgeon as captain of this tight ship. No room for democracy in the operating theatre! The ritual of scrubbing up and the laying on of drapes is like some druidical ceremony. Even the colours of the brilliant carmine red of the arterial blood against the green of the drapes are aesthetically pleasing on the eye. Finally no operation is complete until the wound is neatly dressed and the whole area clean and sparkling again. Just like my desktop at the end of the day.

This love of symmetry and order extends to the way I view my very existence. For example the urge to write this book was not as an ego trip but as a way of achieving closure on the penultimate chapter of my life following my retirement from the NHS and my chair of surgery. However an even more perfect example of my search for one of life's symmetries was provided by chance in 2001 with an invitation to speak at a conference in Warsaw, precisely 100 years after my father's birth in that city.

I was warmly greeted at the airport by two of my hosts. I responded with equal warmth, not sure if I had met them before. What's to lose? Part of the problem of being a minor "celebrity" on the lecture circuit is that you meet thousands of folk on standing down from the podium and, with the best will in the world, you may remember faces and even names, but to put the two together especially when disorientated by foreign travel is beyond my competence. Curiously my wife has that gift but on this occasion she wasn't there to help me out. The day was overcast and grey with a threat of snow and my spirits sank as I was driven through ugly grey suburbs laid out on a bleak flat landscape. My hotel was aesthetically challenged and my room, the best available for the visiting "celebrity", was as bare and charmless as a student's hostel. There was no chair, the light was missing from a bare wire dangling from the ceiling, the pillow was wafer thin (this did not bode well for someone who suffers from reflux oesophagitis), there was no plug in the sink and the soap provided was the size and shape of an After Eight mint. At last, I thought, I'm appearing in a David Lodge campus novel. I revived my spirits a little with a slug of cask strength Glenfarclas I'd wisely bought at Heathrow and consoled myself by thinking that at least on this occasion my wife wasn't with me to whinge. Things could only get better, and they did. That evening I was driven into the old centre of the city for dinner. Next to Sao Paolo in Brazil, Warsaw is the ugliest city I've visited. It consists mainly of grey cube-like apartments that we have come to associate with the workers' paradise of the former Soviet Union. The only building of note as you enter the downtown area is the huge tower of the People's Palace of Culture, a gift from Stalin to the workers of Poland. The grandiose overbearing tower, that looks as if it was built from giant size Lego blocks, is typical of the Stalinist architecture of the 1950s and is an affront to the artistic eye. My Polish hosts were clearly embarrassed by it, as they seemed to be with any discussion of the Soviet period of their history. Things started to get better as we left our cars in the old central square and made our way to the evening's venue. Now it must be remembered that before Warsaw fell to the Russians, the Germans razed it to the ground. In one of the most ignoble episodes of the Second World War, the Russians stood by on the East bank of the Vistula, whilst allowing the Nazis to crush the Polish uprising, in order to allow the leadership of the resistance movement to be liquidated without having to do it themselves. This destruction included the beautiful 16th Century buildings in the central zone, which has now been painstakingly restored to its original appearance. This has been done with such skill that there is no suggestion of an EPCOT-like theme park; it truly looks old. The restaurant was in the barrel-roofed cellar of an old town house full of character and charm, as was my dinner companion Dr. Anna Niwinska, although she was a lot younger. Two glasses of special vodka later I was becoming animated, pledging fraternal toasts to my right and my left.

Two more glasses and I was becoming maudlin telling everyone within earshot about the suffering of my late father as a boy in Warsaw, tearfully asking if it would be possible to visit his birthplace on the meagre information I could supply.

Then the food came in, which I instantly recognized as my late mother's cuisine. Heavy dumplings in barley soup, calf's foot jelly, *cholent* simmered for 24 hours and noodle with raisin pudding for desert. I felt full of contentment and bittersweet memories of my lovely mother who devoted her life to her family, preparing meals like an angel only to die a painful death from breast cancer at the very age I sit writing. After a few more vodka toasts the world went a little fuzzy at the edges and the next morning I woke to find that my slippers were not in their right place.

After two strong cups of coffee I prepared myself for the main event. I was first to chair a session and then, aided by simultaneous translation, to deliver a keynote lecture on my latest clinical research together with philosophical musings on the nature of conceptual models of disease. This seemed to go down well although my witticisms seemed to lose something in translation. I also avoided falling into the trap of patronizing my eastern European audience. For a start the chairman of my session, Professor Jacek Jassem from Gdansk, was President of the European Breast Cancer Conference that year and Marie Curie had started her pioneering work on radium just round the corner. In fact one of the most wonderful products of the fall of the Soviet Empire is the welcoming of many nations with a great scientific tradition back into the bosom of the international scientific community. (Figure 3)

The standard of the meeting as a whole was worthy of their heritage and their hospitality overwhelming. The rest of the meeting fell into a pattern, which I had long come to recognize and enjoy. Speakers dinner the first night, a typical folklorist show the second and the inevitable "gala dinner" and dancing on the last.

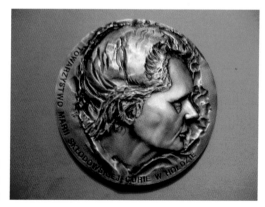

Fig. 3 Marie Curie medal presented on my visit to Warsaw

The show was somewhat unusual – entitled "Musicale, Ach te Musicale" at the Teatrze Roma. It consisted of excerpts from popular musicals translated into Polish.

"My Fair Lady" was a hoot with something definitely lost in translation during the "I'm getting married in the morning" song which came out sounding like "Orang- ootang murdered in the bath tub" but that didn't stop me singing along with the cast. But the next number stopped me in my tracks and had me blubbing into my handkerchief. On came Tevya from "Fiddler on the Roof" to sing, "If I was a rich man da –da- da- da- da –da- da- daya". He was bearded and dressed in a garb seen in the sepia photographs of my paternal grandfather. So here I was, a Londoner in Warsaw, watching a Polish translation of an American musical that was meant to be an evocation of the stetl (village) life from which my family escaped, first to the big city of Warsaw and then to London. Would my grandfather have been proud? I doubt it because along the way I had shed the mantle of the Chassidic Jew and was here in a completely secular role.

The next day of lectures and debates was followed by the "Gala dinner". After the food and the toasts, I went easy on the vodka this time; the joint began to jump to the beat of rhythm and blues. To start with I watched wistfully from the sidelines as the pretty young doctors and their young bucks took to the floor and boogied to the beat. I love dancing and used to be quite good, in fact I won the Mister Twister competition in 1961 whilst a house officer at the Birmingham General Hospital. Perhaps feeling sorry for me a gorgeous blonde medical oncologist dragged me on to the floor and I boogied with the best of them. Suddenly I had a rare moment of self-revelation and saw myself as a sad, rotund, past his sell-by date old professor. I took my leave and went early to bed – the bitter self-revelation, the alcohol and rich food combined with the flat pillow guaranteeing a night of heartburn and insomnia.

My last day in Warsaw was given over to sightseeing and on this occasion my guides were the same Dr. Anna Niwinska and Professor Andrzej Kulakowski, director of the Maria Sklodowska-Curie Memorial Cancer Centre. Professor Kulakowski was born in 1929 and served with the Polish resistance during the uprising in 1943–44. As a boy of 14 he ran backwards and forwards delivering ammunition to the besieged fighters, narrowly missing death on many occasions. He went on to become Poland's leading surgical oncologist. The first stop on my tour was Marie Curie's office to view her memorabilia and to be presented with a memorial medal. After that we made the pilgrimage to the memorial of the Warsaw Ghetto uprising, a noble and awe–inspiring monument raised by the Poles in admiration for the heroism of the Jewish fighters. One of the few survivors was a baby girl smuggled out in a shoebox. I met her a few years ago at a charity event in Frankfurt. She is the wife of the President of the vibrant young Jewish community there. I offered up my prayers and shed a few more tears, becoming more lachrymose by the minute. I was then taken to the Saxony gardens mentioned in my father's memoirs and finally as a coup de grace to the environs of my father's birthplace. Much to my delight and great surprise Anna had taken note of my vodka-fuelled ramblings of the first night and together with Professor Kulakowski, who knew the city like the back of his hand both before and after its destruction, were able to carry out some detective work. With the aid of an old map they had traced the junction of Genshe Street described to me by my father to an area that used to be in the Ghetto. The only building left standing after the Nazis had finished was the Church of the Nativity of the Virgin Mary. After the Russians had moved in they rebuilt the area retaining the old grid of roads, with brutal concrete apartments. The roads were renamed after Soviet heroes. Standing at the corner of Anielewicza and Karlmelika we ran out of clues and were about to leave it at that when a bent old babushka of 80 plus years emerged from her ground floor flat. She had total recall of the topography of that area, having served nearby as a maid in the pre-war years. Her claw-like hand took mine and dragged me one block away where she pointed "Genshe, Genshe!" I gave her all my zlotys and with my mobile phoned my oldest brother Geoffrey to tell him that I had traced our roots. Roots schmoots! If my grandfather hadn't taken the initiative to leave Warsaw in 1912 I wouldn't be here today, but at least my need for symmetry was satisfied.

Chapter 2

The Simple Son

"Then the simple son enquired
What should Passover mean to me?
To which his father replied
You were freed from slavery"
The Haggadah

I was born in the East End of London on May 31st 1937 at 12.00 noon, the day of the Grand National. My father often told the story of his little flutter on the race. He was torn between "Royal Mail" and "Midday Sun" and chose the latter partly because of his left wing tendency and partly because his third son was born at midday. Royal Mail won the race at 100/6 whilst Midday Sun broke a leg and had to be shot. I was not amused by this story and felt it as a bad omen, starting life with an inferiority complex. This was not helped by the fact that I was the third of four sons. On the eves of the first and second days of Passover all Jews celebrate the *Seder* night, where we read out the story of the exodus from Egypt. The master of the house conducts the service from a beautifully illustrated book, the Haggadah. As well as the narrative, the service is interspersed with the eating of foods rich in symbolism, nursery songs to keep the youngsters awake, ritual debates and homilies. Amongst the latter is the tale of the four sons. One is wise, the second wicked, the third simple and the fourth too young to understand. Each is given the task of questioning the leader of the service on the meaning of the festivities. In the tradition of our family each son had to act the part according to seniority. My eldest brother Geoffrey was the wise son, my brother Harold the wicked, me the simple and the youngest David as the "child who does not know how to ask". My lines were easy to learn all I had to say was "what is all this then?" What started as simple play-acting fed a growing understanding that I was indeed the simple one in the family as well as the one doomed to fall at the first fence. Surprisingly, I never resented this role, which soon became a self-fulfilling prophecy, and took great consolation from the achievements of my siblings. (Figure 4)

It was only when I became a senior academic that I began to appreciate the importance of the naive question, "what is all this then?" and "how do we know?"

Before I tell you about my family and upbringing I want to try to give a flavour of life in England in the mid to late 1930s. To do this I've drawn on my earliest memories, family folklore, and from a series of Punch magazines of 1937 that I bought in a car boot sale. (Figures 5, 6, 7) England in the late 1930s was at a transition

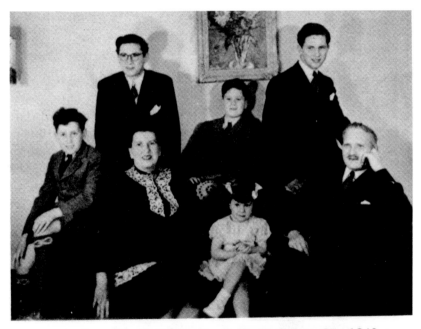

The family at 39 Sandon Road, Birmingham–circa 1948.
From left to right: the boys: David, Harold, Michael, Geoffrey
On the settee: Mum, Linda, Dad

Fig. 4 Picture of my family when I was about 11

between Edwardian values and Modernism. This was well illustrated by the graphic art In Punch at this time. At one extreme we see the classicism of Bernard Partridge whilst at the other the extreme simplicity of line by Fougasse. It is also immediately apparent that every household had servants who are illustrated in cartoons of either self-satire or what would now be considered most politically incorrect, mockery of the servant class. The first might include that famous series by Pont, lampooning the British Character. In one captioned "Love of never throwing anything away", we see a uniformed maid looking in despair at the clutter in the attic. In another captioned "Absence of ideas for meals" it is the mistress of the house who holds her head in despair whilst cook waits impassively. As far as the second category is concerned this exchange appears below a meticulous drawing of madam addressing the maid. "Mary, your mother has just telephoned to say your sister has flu". "Flew, Madam? But where has she went?" Funny thing is, although I grew up in a family that appeared to be penniless, we always had a maid. The maid was always from Ireland as I recall and mother had to "let one go" because she had a crush on my brother Geoff. In Punch of that time middle class men sported bristly moustaches, wore hats and spats and smoked Craven "A", made specially "to prevent sore throats". My father could have been the stereotype for the protagonists in this one. "Hallo, old man, I thought you were on a diet". "Ah, I had my diet at home before I came to the club". Yet behind this veneer of jolly

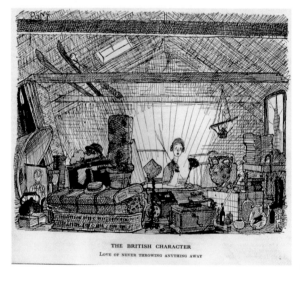

THE BRITISH CHARACTER
LOVE OF NEVER THROWING ANYTHING AWAY

Fig. 5 Punch cartoon from the mid 1930s

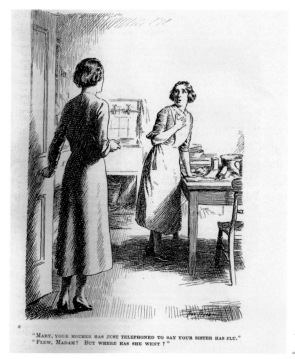

Fig. 6 Punch cartoon from the mid 1930s

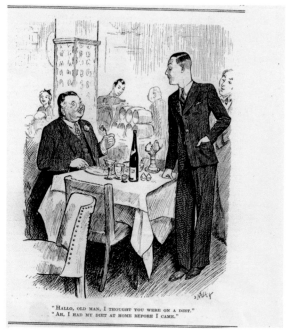

Fig. 7 Punch cartoon from the mid 1930s

old England, Punch was sensitive to the early signs of the gathering storm. In one cartoon that I still find funny, we see the House of Commons with all the members wearing gas masks. ("Gas drill at Westminster") One MP is on his feet addressing the house declaiming, "And I think I may confidently say, judging from the expressions on the faces of the honourable members, that the house is in unanimous agreement with the views I have expressed". Clearly then as now the public were afraid of enemies who might attack with chemical and biological weapons. (Figure 8) Another more sombre in tone reminds us of the anti-war faction in the UK before Hitler invaded Poland. We see Sir Stafford Cripps standing on a soapbox ranting away whilst in the background we see darkening clouds and a sky full of bombers labelled "Foreign Menace". The caption reads, "Today you have the most glorious opportunity that the workers have ever had...refuse to make munitions, refuse to make armaments."

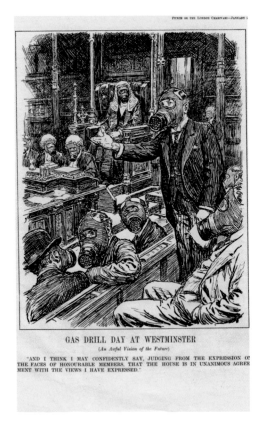

GAS DRILL DAY AT WESTMINSTER
(An Awful Vision of the Future)

"AND I THINK I MAY CONFIDENTLY SAY, JUDGING FROM THE EXPRESSION OF THE FACES OF HONOURABLE MEMBERS, THAT THE HOUSE IS IN UNANIMOUS AGREEMENT WITH THE VIEWS I HAVE EXPRESSED."

Fig. 8 Punch cartoon from the mid 1930s

In fact my first, albeit fragmented memories, are of the blitz round about 1941/42 when I must have been about four or five. I remember the sirens followed by the night-time rush to the Anderson shelter that my father and helpers had dug in the garden. I wasn't frightened but because of the competition to get on the top bunk I rushed out ahead of the family and slipped down the rain-slicked step of our bunker. I remember the steel re-enforced kitchen table that served as a shelter if the alarm hadn't sounded before the first bomb fell. My two older brothers would scoop up their books or schoolwork and carry on reading under the table barely missing a beat. Because of the blitz my father moved the family from the East End of London to Birmingham and when the bombers followed us there, to Halesowen in the Midlands . There I remember being held up at a window to see Coventry in flames as the Germans bombed it to hell. There was no hiding the little ones in the industrial cities any more so for a short time we became evacuees in a Welsh farming community. I must have been very unhappy there because ever since I've had an aversion to the country although I love the Welsh.

At the end of the war when I was 7 or 8 my father moved us back to Birmingham, from when my coherent memories begin. We lived in a large rambling Edwardian house at the corner of Sandon Road and City Road in Edgbaston. Not long afterwards the first premonition of a new addition to the family occurred when a starling flew into the scullery where my mother was washing up. Summoned by her screams, I was to learn that according to family legend each Baum pregnancy was signalled by a bird flying into the house. Furthermore all Baum children are born with a bird shaped birth-mark on their back. Indeed I have a birth mark on my back that could just about be interpreted as a bird with folded wings, but the symbolism of all this escaped me and only added to my sense of insecurity, suggesting once again that my fate was pre-determined. Six months later, with much rejoicing, my baby sister Linda was born. My mother was about 40 at that time but she and my father were desperate to have a daughter (Girls are a rare commodity in my family and of my 9 grandchildren only one is of the female gender.)

As already mentioned my father was a very handsome and dapper gentleman who served in Dad's Army (The Home Guard) during the war with great distinction; putting out incendiary bombs with a stirrup pump and going on manoeuvres with live ammunition, to my mother's profound alarm. Fortunately the West Midlands never saw German parachutists and the nearest he came to the enemy was when a Messerschmitt crash-landed in a neighbouring field, with the pilot still in the cockpit. My Dad's daytime job was as a special agent. Until I was brutally enlightened I always thought that he was a spy like "Dick Barton-Special Agent" the hero of a popular radio serial drama. Sadly his work was neither glamorous nor rewarding. He wasn't an agent of the state but an agent of the *schmutter* business, *schmutter* being Yiddish for rags. In other words he sold women's dresses to the high street retailers. I learnt of his daily humiliations the hard way when eventually joining him as a helper on his daily rounds during the long summer holidays. I remember how he was patronized or kept waiting by the "all-important" buyers for the lady's gown departments of the local Midlands towns. Here was a man with no formal education beyond the age of 11, with parents who only spoke Yiddish, and sadly no flare for or patience with the world of commerce. Condemned to a lifelong struggle to finance a large and hungry family he yet managed to educate himself through his voracious appetite for books. He was clearly a very intelligent man, representing the City of Birmingham at bridge and chess. He could play 12 boards simultaneously and win them all blindfolded. Apart from these activities he fought hard for some kind of self-esteem via the Masonic Lodge and the Hebrew Community. He went on to become Worshipful Master of his Lodge and represented the Birmingham Jewish Community on the Board of Deputies of British Jewry. Sadly this lead to many rows between my parents as his business suffered through neglect. In the end like many of his generation he looked towards his children to benefit from the advantages of living in a free, liberal and democratic nation that of course included a free and liberal education.

In the meantime, unrecognized until many years later, the central component of my education was already fixed in place by the ubiquity of books cluttering the house and the passionate dialectic of the family debates around the Friday night dinner table. It must have been here that I learnt to see the "other hand" of the "on the one hand but on the other hand" duality. It must have been here that I learnt to enjoy defending the indefensible just for the hell of it. Apart from the ritual of the *Erev Shabbat* I enjoyed a reasonably strict orthodox Jewish upbringing. This meant walking about three miles to the Birmingham Singer's Hill Synagogue every Saturday morning and sitting through endless sermons. It also meant attending all the festivals, most of which congregated round the beginning of each new school term, which didn't help my secular education. At the age of 13 I was *Bar Mitzvahed*. By all accounts I had a beautiful singing voice before puberty and I had the congregation in tears with my readings from the Torah Scroll and the Prophets. The most memorable event on that day was the cheque I received from my rich, flamboyant and philandering uncle Sid. It was made out for £13.12s.6p, a princely if somewhat mysterious sum for those days. Later it emerged that he got his cheques mixed up and this one should have gone to his turf accountant. Instead I got a large white 5 pound note the size of a handkerchief, which somehow felt more valuable than the cheque, not that it mattered as my father pocketed all the monetary gifts to pay for the function. But at least I got to keep the fountain pens. I never found out what a turf accountant was but from the hushed tones of my parents I suspected it was something dirty. From the age of 13 I was meant to fulfil all the religious duties of an adult Jew and every so often my paternal grandfather would descend on the household, with the vengeance and appearance of an Old Testament prophet, to check up on the minutiae of my observance. Things got a little better when suddenly, at the age of 13½, I noticed that there were girls sitting in the upstairs gallery. I then realized that as we had a *mixed* choir and I had a good voice then religious observance wouldn't be too tiresome if I joined the choir.

My oldest brother Geoff was the first in the family to go to University. He qualified in medicine in 1955 and started off as a gallant captain in the RAMC in Egypt before settling into a successful career as a general practitioner. He was also a first class rugby player, a member of Moseley RFC and a county triallist. How he managed this is still a mystery to me. In fact the opportunity provided by this book allows me to confess, after a lifetime in denial, one dark secret, one missed opportunity, which has haunted me all my life. My regret concerns rugby football. I love rugby football and think it's the best spectator sport of all but I didn't always want to be a spectator; I wanted to be a player. I wasn't ambitious enough to want to score the last minute drop goal that allowed England to beat the All Blacks or even play for the Wasps; I only wanted to play for my school's first XV. Of course I wasn't big enough to play in the pack, or fast enough to play on the wing, but I was sufficiently nimble and quick-witted to have made a useful scrum half. So what stopped me? Well as already mentioned I grew up in an orthodox Jewish household and *Shabbat* was devoted to the synagogue and quiet study. Saturday was also the day for rugby practice and matches of our school XV. Even if I slipped away in the afternoon on a pretext, I was so full of *cholent,* the traditional Sabbath hot pot, that there was not enough blood left to flow to my legs, as most of my circulation was diverted to my gastro-intestinal tract. So I regret all that time spent in the synagogue, praying in a language I didn't understand, listening to boring sermons and eating heavy midday meals, when I could have been playing scrum half for the school and who knows, even for my medical school.

But then there is a law of unintended consequences. I might have suffered brain damage, left the fold, and missed out on that occasion when I met my current wife. The sliding doors of life might then have left me at 70 as a lonely grumpy old man without a woman to call his own and without 9 adorable grandchildren.

Next in seniority was my brother Harold. He was extremely gifted academically and was something of a prodigy at school. He went on to become Professor of biochemistry and Dean of life science at King's College London. It was through him that I discovered the meaning of the scientific process and the thirst for discovery. He is still a great lyricist and famous for writing the Biochemists' Songbook.

My youngest brother David "crept up from behind" to win every prize, including the rarely minted gold medal, on qualifying in medicine at Birmingham University three years after me in 1963. He enjoyed a spectacular career rising to become Professor of Paediatrics and Child Health at Bristol University and then President of his Royal College. He died at the age of 59 literally whilst in the saddle, leading a charity bike ride to raise money to support the health care needs of child victims of the Balkan wars. He taught me the meaning of hard work, vision and self-belief.

The youngest of us all was our beloved little sister who went on to serve the NHS as a hard working underpaid speech therapist. When she followed my mother with a diagnosis of breast cancer at the age of 45 my world turned over and my mission shifted from career development for its own sake to one fuelled by a fire in my belly to rid the world of breast cancer. What sheer bloody arrogance and conceit you might think, and rightly so, yet my youngest brother (Figure 9) set out to change the world of childhood suffering and died in the attempt. He always illustrated his attitude with the parable of the star-fish.

An old man walking on the beach at dawn noticed a boy picking up a starfish and throwing it into the sea. When asked why, the boy explained that the stranded starfish would die if left to lie in the morning sun. 'But there are millions of starfish on

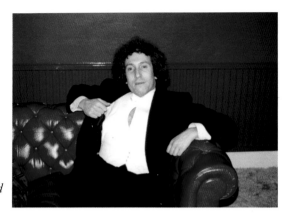

Fig. 9 My brother David in his prime

this beach,' said the old man. 'How can your efforts make a difference?' The boy picked up another starfish and placed it in the waves. 'It makes a difference to this one,' he said.

Little guys like us can change the world a little for the better if we all have high ambitions and are willing to fail triumphantly.

However it was a long and rocky road to develop that self-belief and shake off my childish notion of being the simple son. The nadir of my academic achievements was when I became bottom of the class in a third rate grammar school in Birmingham. My father feigned delight and explained that I would be looked after if I left school at 16 and joined him in business. The thought of this living hell, as experienced whilst helping out in my summer holidays, galvanized me into action. I gained reasonable results at GCSE O levels and then surprised my family and myself by gaining a state scholarship that allowed me to follow my brothers into Birmingham University in 1955.

As much as I hated grammar school, I loved medical school. I loved the camaraderie around the cadaver on the anatomy dissecting table, I loved the patient contact on the medical firms, I loved the drama of A&E and the operating theatre, but most of all I loved the rugger-bugger beer-swilling parties and the *goyisher* (gentile) girls at the Saturday night hops. Up until that time I'd never really drunk anything other than the sacramental *kiddush* wine on Friday night and Passover. Furthermore my relationship with the girls of the Jewish youth societies and study groups was decorous, inhibited by an intense shyness and consummated only by a fierce game of table tennis. Even the chance mention of a girl's name at the family

Friday night dinner was enough to make me blush to the roots of my hair and leave the table in confusion. Ah, but medical school and my two years "in house" as a resident medical officer were heaven (as long as my parents didn't find out!). I qualified as a doctor in 1960 with relative ease, enjoyed my appointment as house surgeon at my teaching hospital, the Queen Elizabeth Hospital Birmingham, and experienced the excitement and instant gratification as a senior house officer in A & E at the Birmingham General Hospital. I passed my primary FRCS (Fellow of the Royal College of Surgeons) studying in my spare time, and was all set for a career in surgery when I was overtaken by Zionistic zeal whilst (ahem) simultaneously escaping from an inappropriate relationship. In the spring of 1963 I approached the Jewish agency in Tel Aviv and in no time at all found myself on the SS Theodore Herzl, out of Marseilles en route to Haifa.

Chapter 3

In the steps of Josephus
Israel 1963–1964

I am British by accident of birth thanks to the fact that both my sets of grandparents escaped the pogroms in Russia and Poland, by fleeing to London early in the last century. This country has been good to our family, providing us with free health care and a free education that allowed my generation to reach the highest levels of academia. My youngest brother David ended his life as President of the Royal College of Paediatrics and Child Health (RCPCH). As mentioned earlier he died tragically at the age of 59 whilst leading a charity bike ride for the children of Kosovo, and is buried in Rosh Pinah overlooking the Sea of Galilee in Northern Israel. His will and his family's choice of this burial site reflect the spiritual pull of Israel for many Western Jews. His last act was to establish a children's clinic in Gaza for the training of Palestinian doctors. This project amongst others is continued by the RCPCH in the name of the David Baum International Fund (DBIF). This act also reflects the Jewish angst about the suffering of the Palestinians.

In May 2004 I was a guest of the University in Haifa, along with a small faculty from the USA, for a workshop on the prevention of cancer. Cancer epidemiology is one of the strengths in Israeli medical research. The Israeli population is an extraordinary mix of ethnic types who retain the majority of their genetic and cultural distinctions. This provides an almost unique "natural experiment" for the study of the contributions of both nature and nurture to the risk of developing breast cancer. On the one hand we have the Ashkenazi and Sephardi Jews with similar cultures but striking difference in their risk of inheritance of mutations for the breast cancer predisposition (BRCA) genes (see chapter 14). On the other hand we have the village dwelling and nomadic Arab (Bedouin) populations with similar genetic pools but very different life styles. There are also the Christian Arabs, Bahai and Druze. As well as their different risk factors, their different cultures and life styles provide unique problems for screening and management of the disease. Israeli academics have exploited these opportunities in a way that informs the rest of the world.

Haifa is a beautiful city dominated by the Bahai temple and gardens occupying the slopes of Mount Carmel. l warmly approve of the Bahai belief system because of its tolerance and universal appeal. The Bahais elected to set up their HQ in Haifa because, as a breakaway sect of Islam, they were persecuted in all Islamic countries. For hundreds of years the Arab and Jewish population have got on well in Haifa, with many joint projects and an Arab mayor quite recently. This peaceful co-existence was shattered by the second intifada.

From Haifa we were driven down the axis of the country just to the west of the new barrier that separates the *disputed territories* from Israel proper. Along 95% of its length is a wire fence with electronic surveillance devices, the remainder is made up of an ugly concrete wall that is commonly seen in the media worldwide. No one mentions that this has been built to stop snipers firing on traffic on the A6 motorway from high-rise apartments that overlook the road. I have little doubt that some sections of the wall have caused hardship, and a recent appeal by Palestinians to the Israeli high court was successful, with the result that sections of the wall will be re-routed. If there were any Jews left in Arab lands I can't imagine the reverse holding true, but then they were all expelled after the 1948 war, a silent 800,000 that the world press never acknowledges. The fence works and the terrorist atrocities in Northern Israel have been stifled.

Having reached Beer-Sheba we turned east to the Dead Sea. Along the way we saw many new villages housing the Bedouin tribes. Their romantic nomadic life was in fact brutal and short and although they maintain all their traditions of hospitality in their black tents, their health and quality of life has been improved by settling them on pasture-land with free schooling and health care. The Bedu are loyal Israeli citizens and even serve in the Israel Defence Force (IDF).

The ride down to the Dead Sea never fails to strike awe in my heart but the effect is then spoiled when you arrive at the luxury hotels at Ein Bokkek close to the biblical site of Sodom. Here the visiting faculty spoke to a conference of about 200 Israeli and Arab doctors. My role was to discuss the pros and cons of screening for breast and prostate cancer. After the meeting a group of us travelled 20 km north to Massada, the famous archaeological site that marks Herod's winter palace and the last stand of the Jewish resistance to the Roman occupation after the destruction of the second temple in 70CE.

On this barren plateau (Figure 10) 1,000 metres above the Dead Sea the view looking east to the mountains of Moab is breathtaking. You can still see the Roman siege wall and pray in the oldest synagogue in the world. You may know the story of how, after a three year siege, the 900 survivors committed suicide rather than surrender to the Romans who persecuted them because of their faith. For this reason Massada has become a symbol of resistance in Israel and the graduation ceremony for certain brigades of the IDF takes place on

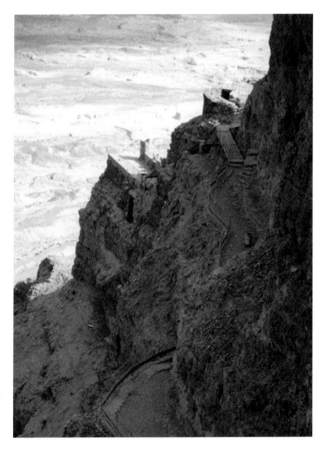

Fig. 10 King Herod's Palace at the northern edge of Masada

21

Massada, where they pledge, *"Shaynit M'zada Lo Tipol",* Massada will not fall a second time. I find this kind of heroic militarism embarrassing, (after all I never let my kids and grandchildren play with guns and toy tanks), but we in the U.K. enjoy a guaranteed security, apart from the odd threat of an IRA or Al Qaida bomb. In Israel though this pledge to self-defence is not paranoia, because for more than 50 years the combined armies of Syria, Jordan, Iraq, Iran and Egypt have made various attempts at taking Massada a second time. Fortunately Egypt and Jordan have negotiated peace whilst Iraq has other problems on its mind at the moment.

At the base of the mountain is a beautiful new museum that describes the archaeological history of the area and the history of its excavation. In the latter section I was startled and almost moved to tears to see a picture of myself aged 27, (see Figure 11) resplendent in a chequered keffiya and a red beard from the time I was acting as deputy medical officer on the dig during the winter season 1963/64.

Shortly after gaining my primary FRCS whilst working in the A & E department of the Birmingham General Hospital, I went to work in Israel. I was motivated by a lust for adventure, a need for surgical experience in the field and as a visionary Zionist. According to the new left wing ideology, Zionism is a dirty word stigmatised by the infamous UN resolution that equated Zionism with Racism in 1971. In contrast the Zionist movement is merely an expression of the Jewish people's yearning to find security in a land they can call their own after two millennia of persecution. Even amongst my own friends and family who have grown up in this country and never experienced a whiff of anti-Semitism, I detect paranoia in our dinner party conversations. Mostly this is due to a vestigial folk sub-consciousness, but more recently this has been fuelled by the unholy alliance of the extreme left wing media and the fundamentalists amongst our Islamic population.

There are secular and religious Zionists who may be right wing or left wing. I would classify myself as of the left-leaning secular variety. The accusation that Zionism is an expression of racism and apartheid can be refuted simply by noting the treatment of the Bedu described above and my first hand experience described below.

In the spring of 1963 I packed all my worldly belongings in one suitcase, closed my bank account, taking the balance of £70 as my only asset, and made my way down south to Marseilles. There I boarded the Theodore Herzl and for three days sailed east to the Promised Land. As Mount Carmel and Haifa emerged out of the early morning haze there wasn't a dry eye amongst those making *aliyah* (literally translated as making the ascent but now translated as immigration) who crowded the bow deck. From Haifa I made my way to Tel-Aviv and the offices of the Jewish Agency with whom I had been conducting my affairs and from whom I had been promised a job as a junior surgeon in the newly opened teaching hospital in Beer-Sheba. That was where my troubles began. This utterly incompetent and bureaucratic organization had no knowledge of my existence, the job did not exist and the hospital was still on the drawing board. I found temporary accommodation in a hostel for English speaking immigrants, Bet Brodedsky in Ramat Aviv, just North of Tel Aviv, and set out to find work. I blew most of my savings on a second hand Vespa and wasted a week queuing in the dusty heat at a series of departments that controlled traffic regulations, to get my driving licence. Thus my first disillusionments with the Zionist dream were stimulated by my first experience of the infamous bureaucracy of this new democratic nation.

That aside I was elated by the sense of devil-may-care freedom from all responsibilities, the wind in my hair in the heat of a beautiful Israeli spring, and the thrill of my first ascent to the golden city of Jerusalem. The elation didn't last long as first I was hit full in the face by the *chumsin,* the hot dry wind that blows off the Arabian peninsula sporadically at that time of year and is known to drive people into a homicidal frenzy, and secondly by the problem of finding a job. Naively I had assumed that the world was waiting for me: this brilliant young English surgeon with half an FRCS under his belt. In reality I found out that there was an overabundance of doctors in Israel, the heads of departments were mostly German refugees who didn't rate the FRCS and finally my rudimentary command of *Ivrit,* (modern Hebrew), was considered a disadvantage. Even if I spoke English very slowly and loudly it didn't help my case. Like most Jewish boys I learnt biblical Hebrew at *cheder,* (Sunday school). I could read from the prayer books and sight-read the melodies from the encrypted notation in the *Chumash,* the books of the Torah and Prophets. This was only of limited value for me for the following reasons: the pronunciation was different, the writing of Modern Hebrew lacks vowels and there were no words for cholecystectomy or achlorhydria. I was as much use in the surgical outpatient department in Israel as Beowulf would be in the NHS A&E department. Eventually I became quite fluent in *ivrit* from a combination of evening classes and learning on the job. Although to begin with my chat-up line on first (and usually last) dates with Israeli nurses was limited to polite enquiry as to the regularity of their bowel and menstrual function. With even greater experience and fluency I ventured into the territory of urinary frequency and abdominal cramps. I was also in deep trouble in the operating theatre because the words for scissors, trousers and spectacles sounded almost alike to my untrained ear. Imagine asking for a sharp pair of trousers when trying to cut through dense fibrous tissue in a case of diverticulitis! Joking aside this experience taught me what it must be like to be new immigrants in the UK from the Indian subcontinent who suffer humiliations and ridicule because of their failure to master the English language. This must have been how my Yiddish speaking grandparents felt 100 years ago.

Eventually I was posted to a large community hospital in Afula serving the Jezreal valley and caring for the needs of a mixed bunch of secular Jewish Kibbutzniks, Religious Jews from S'fad, Moslem Arabs from the local villages and Christian Arabs from Nazareth; an exotic brew of folk who were all treated with equal respect or occasionally equal rudeness! Many of the doctors were Arabs trained in Israel and there was some intermarriage on the campus.

In spite of my early difficulties I learnt much of lifelong value in the subjects of surgical techniques and human relationships. My mentor and head of department was Professor Shmuel Nissan, recently in post after having been chief resident in an American teaching hospital. He was a tall, handsome and rugged character, who had been born into an old established Jewish Palestinian family, veterans of the first *aliyah.* A multi-cultured man, he was fluent in Arabic as well as English and Ivrit and was popular amongst the elders of some of the local Arab villages. He grew citrus fruit on his farm and raised Arab horses and was also a medical historian. He ultimately went on to become chief of surgery at the Mount Scopus branch of the Hadassah hospital in Jerusalem. He taught me how to do a *real* radical mastectomy – the American Halsted technique. (See chapter 6)

Apart from learning the skills of elective surgery I had my share of emergency work. Being in essentially a rural community I remember a number of grisly accidents with tractors. More important than this was my modest yet informative introduction into the management of gunshot wounds. Although 1963–65 was a relatively peaceful time in the history of Israel there were still feddayin raids and sniper fire from the Golan Heights, aimed at farmers in the fertile Beit Shan valley below. There was one extraordinary incident when I had to deal with two soldiers shot with one bullet as they patrolled the border. The sniper had managed to pierce the hand of the nearest and the shoulder of the second as they rode together in a comradely pose. On that occasion I had to give evidence to the blue berets of the UN soldiers monitoring the peace. There were hundreds of such incidents each year.

My next adventure was being sent to help out the Scottish Mission Hospital in Nazareth when their only surgeon was on sick leave. I loved the nuns who made up the nursing staff and admired their strict discipline that was in stark contrast to the laissez faire democratic attitude of the Israeli nurses in the *kupat cholim* (workers fund) hospital in Afula. The nuns acted as interpreters in the clinics and as surgical assistants in the theatre. By this time I was fairly proficient in the standard elective and emergencies but there was one occasion I operated with a book held up in front of me. One night a baby was born with an open spina bifida, a congenital defect where the spinal column fails to fuse over the spinal cord. With the spinal cord exposed, infection and meningitis would be inevitable and the nearest hospital with a paediatric surgeon was two hours away. Learning on the job I completed the task of mobilizing the delicate membranes around the spinal canal and succeeded in closing the defect. The baby survived but for all I knew went on to develop other complications linked to this congenital abnormality. From my current standpoint I shudder to think of my hubris at the time but I felt good about myself then, and a pretty young nun made me hot chocolate before I collapsed exhausted into my bed, (which I sometimes shared with a pair of friendly geckoes!).

That aside my biggest adventure was being sent as deputy medical officer to the Massada dig…

Shmuel Nissan was the nephew of the President of the State of Israel, Zalman Shazar. He in turn was a close friend of Professor Yigal Yadin who was chief of staff of the IDF during the 1948 war of independence and as a second career went on to become professor of archaeology at the Hebrew University in Jerusalem. He was in charge of the excavations of King Herod's palace at Massada. Thus through a complex series of interactions, known in Israel as *protectia,* I was invited to volunteer as deputy medical officer at the dig. One early morning in February 1963, I started my great adventure by bouncing along un-surfaced tracks in a military jeep driving due east from the desert town of Arad to the foot of the mountain plateau dominating the western shore of the Dead Sea midway between the salt works at S'dom (remember Lot's wife?) and the oasis of Ein Gedi where King

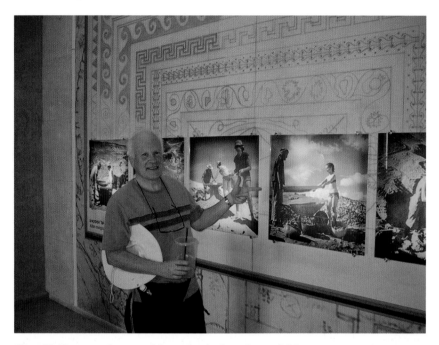

Fig. 11 Picture of me at Massada Archaeological Museum

David hid in a cave from a vengeful King Saul. The archaeologist's encampment was arranged just north west of the remains of the Roman camp where Flavius Silva commanded the Roman legions in their three-year siege of the mountain fortress between 70 and 73 CE. The foot of the Roman siege ramp that rose nearly 1,000 feet to the summit separated the modern from the ancient invaders. In 73 CE the Roman foot soldiers and their siege machines stormed the fortifications at the top only to find that the 900 Jewish zealots who had held out there following the sacking of Jerusalem and the destruction of the second temple had committed suicide rather than fall into the hands of their enemies. As an archaeological site it was therefore of extraordinary value in providing insight into two periods of history, King Herod the Roman Viceroy *and* the period after the fall of the second temple.

My accommodation was an army tent with three other volunteers and I shared duties with a mysterious American doctor in his fifties, working in a field hospital tent. Each morning before dawn we would climb to the summit up the Roman ramp to gaze in awe at the sun rising over the mountains of Moab in Jordan, through the early mist rising from the Dead Sea, then glance down a 1,000 foot vertical drop to the salt plains below. Fortunately my medical skills were seldom called upon and I spent most of the time in charge of a small team digging out the debris of nearly two millennia from between the casement walls erected by King Herod to guard his eastern flank. Our interest was in discovering the domestic details of the life of the zealots who set up home in these quarters. Two of the team dug and filled the buckets, I emptied the buckets into a large sieve held and shaken by another two volunteers. As they sieved the rubble and sand I looked for artefacts before the remaining debris was tipped over the edge of the cliff face. This way we found roman pottery shards and glassware shimmering with a fluorescent light in the strong sunshine, miraculously surviving from the time of Christ. Once we had cleared the bulk of the debris we began the careful task of cleaning the floor and searching for the clues of day-to-day life. I personally uncovered a cooking hearth by following down a trail of soot staining the junction of two stone walls. Hidden under a flagstone making up the hearth I uncovered a rotting woven sack containing a congealed mass of bright blue discs. I watched with fascination as one of the professional archaeologists in the camp treated the find with dilute acetic acid following which the long hidden copper coinage revealed itself as new. The faces of the coins showed "the chalice and the pomegranates" marking them out as 73CE. So I found myself handling the loose change of a Jewish mother who had perished 1900 years earlier. The hairs stood up on the nape of my neck and one of the coins happened to "stick to the palm of my hand". Latterly it served as a lucky charm when I sat my exams to become a fellow of the Royal College of Surgeons in 1965.

The other moving experience for me was the celebration of the Jewish New Year for trees. Here we planted palm and myrtle in this long barren place that had once supported 900 souls for over three years and here we prayed in the first synagogue to be built after the destruction of the second temple.

For recreation we would climb down the precipitous serpentine path that wound down the eastern escarpment and go off on rambles to explore the region of Ein Geddi or follow the encircling siege walls built by the Romans and still visible to all.

In the evening we would have lectures from the archaeologists including a memorable one by Professor Yadin himself, describing the finding of the Bar-Kochba caves just South of Qumran. Other evenings I would gather with my senior colleague and two lady friends for Turkish coffee and gossip in the field hospital. I could deduce nothing about the training or provenance of this American doctor but as we packed up to leave a month later he gave me an address just outside Florence suggesting we meet up on my return to England.

A year later I found myself in Italy having landed at the Port of Rome en route home. A minor detour to Florence lead me to the gate in the high wall protecting Villa Marcello Fincino in Fiesoli. (I later learnt that Fincino was one of the leading lights of the Italian renaissance.) I was surprised to be shown into sumptuous gardens by a liveried servant who conducted me to his master sitting on the terrace of the most beautiful 16thC palace you can imagine. My host the mysterious American doctor, my colleague in Massada, owned a chain of private hospitals in the USA, and according to his story was in hiding from hitmen hired by his estranged wife. After a few days of luxury, living the life of a Florentine prince, I returned to England to pick up my career again and search for a wife.

Chapter 4

Fellowship, Rings and King's

I returned to Birmingham expecting a warm welcome from the family and my teaching hospital. Well at least the former were welcoming; once I had shaved off my rather dashing red beard. The latter were frankly indifferent. Yet again I had overestimated my self-worth. My old professor and mentor had unforgivably died during my absence, so I had no choice but to throw myself at the mercy of the back pages of the British Medical Journal. I was short-listed for a rather good training appointment in the West Midlands but never made the interview because the "big ends" on my rather equally dashing red MGA blew up on the motorway. Although I never forgave the friend who sold me that load of junk, it was thanks to him and his rusty cylinders that I eventually met my wife and on that "sliding door" of the instant, the die was cast that eventually determined my future happiness and the very presence of my adored nine grandchildren. The hair on my neck prickles at the thought of a parallel universe where life has not treated me so kindly.

Next on the list of ticks on the BMJ appointment pages was the Newcastle-upon-Tyne General Hospital. This time I went up by train and then took the tram up to the grim and darkening complex of buildings that suggested L.S. Lowry in one of his depressive moods. I could hardly enjoy the euphoria of success when I was offered the post, as it was conditional on being a resident for at least 12 months in what looked like a Victorian prison. Anyway my new colleagues told me that "the lasses were canny, and that I wouldna gai nay time to sit 'yon me backbody laddee bye the bye". (Whatever that meant – bloody foreigners!)

I returned home and loaded up my now roadworthy MGA convertible, (which would in the end justify its existence), and drove through sleet and snow 200 miles north, with my mood and core body temperature falling (the heater failed en route) the nearer I got to Grimsgrey on Tyne. I checked into my garret in the doctor's residence and unpacked my few belongings and the massive pile of books I needed in order to study for my final fellowship of the Royal College of Surgeons (FRCS). Lonely and sad I found my way to the doctor's "mess" for an early supper only to be greeted by a six foot six inch jovial giant, young Miles Irving (later to become Sir Miles Irving, vice President of the RCS and Chairman of the Newcastle Hospitals NHS trust). He had recently joined the staff and along with other jovial young men I was introduced to the mess bar, paid my dues and quickly learnt that living "on the house" in Coaltip on Tees was not quite as bad as I first thought.

The loss of the culture of the resident doctor's mess in a NHS hospital leaves me feeling saddened. In return for free board and lodgings, laundry, and social centre we worked about 11 hours a day and usually were on call one night and one weekend in three. The pay was derisory but we learnt quickly on the job, the patients enjoyed continuity of care and the camaraderie was fantastic. Our only complaint was the very uncertain career development as our "junior doctor" days were open ended, with the hope of a consultant job the light at the end of a very long tunnel. Nowadays, with shift work, European convention on hours of work and a shortened and very structured career development, we have lost the professionalism and continuity of care, and the young consultant is very inexperienced. Of course the bottleneck is now at the transition from registered doctor to a specialist training programme, with much unemployment and emigration. A lot of value has been lost along the way, and morale is at an all time low. The NHS is in a mess; bring back the "mess" to the NHS. (Oh my god I sound like a grumpy old man!)

Once I was settled in, I began studying for the FRCS in my spare time, but needed some leisure activity as well. It would have been easy to slip back into bad habits of wine women and song, but I'd been down that route once and I'd also experienced loneliness for the first time in my life whilst working in rural Israel. So the first free night I had off duty before 8.00pm, I took myself off to Maccabi House, the cultural and sporting centre for young Jewish men and women. I was greeted at the door by a very friendly Geordie lad, (by the way I must say that all the Geordie folk were warm and friendly to me), who wanted to know my business in town. I explained I was there as a surgeon in training who wanted to join in the Jewish cultural and sporting life in Newcastle. He replied as far as I can recall with, "thouserlooken for a wee Jewish Geordie lass, if ah'mm nay mistook". I demurred for a while but he pressed me. "Thar's that bonnie Judy Marcus lass, her's as workin in the Obstreporous department at thar General Ospidal, ard luke her up if a'r waz yoo, she's right friendly like." I found someone to translate for me and at the first opportunity, on a pathetic pretext, I made my way into the department of O&G, making sure to turn up the neck of my white coat and drape my stethoscope casually around my shoulders. Oh so kool, before the concept of kool had been invented. Plan A was to enquire about the whereabouts of the young girl with an ectopic pregnancy that I'd operated on a couple of nights before. Plan A failed as I was left speechless by this vision of loveliness behind the desk with stunning green eyes and a fashionable Vidal Sassoon haircut. After coolly appraising me, the vision was about to speak, I prayed to God that a) she was the said Miss Marcus and b) that she spoke English. God answered in the affirmative on both accounts. Later I was to learn that while all this turmoil was going on inside my head, she was thinking to herself, "Who the hell is this pompous young prig?" Eventually she fell in love with my MGA roadster, bless its rusty heart, but reserved her judgment about me. After this false start we embarked upon a ménage à trois; Judy, the MG and me. About a year later the MG had to be put out of its misery following an unnerving incident when I was overtaken at speed by my offside rear wheel whilst my rear suspension ploughed up the tarmac. I took this as Nature's way of telling me to grow up.

I worked and courted furiously. Courtship involved a break in my studies between supper and 9.00 pm for a coffee and a cuddle, followed by reading and note taking until 1.00 am most nights, appearing at a clinic or an operating session the following morning. Of course one night in three I might never have gone to bed at all. One of my consultants lived so far away that I was mostly left to deal with the emergencies by myself. Good practice for me but I shudder to think of the mistakes I must have made due to my inexperience. Fortunately that kind of thing has changed for the better. After working day and night through the winter and spring of 1964/65 I registered to sit my final FRCS exam in May. Two weeks before that, the other two trainee surgeons on the house who shared the duty roster with me took off for study leave, so that I was left holding the fort all alone. Much to my surprise I found the exam quite easy and when my number was called out by the clerk of the court of examiners from the top of the stairs at the college in Lincoln's Inn Fields, I floated up past all the magnificent portraits of past presidents, to be welcomed as a fellow by Lord Brock and Sir Hedley Atkins. I look at their signatures on my framed diploma above my desk as I write. I floated back to Newcastle on the last train and collapsed exhausted on my bed.

The following morning, without anything being said about my FRCS, my chief addressed me as **Mister** Baum for the first time. The warm glow I experienced on losing the title Dr. is very difficult to explain to lay people. It's all part of the very English inverse snobbery whereby surgeons recall the days of our guild with the Royal Charter being presented by King Henry VIII. Once you had mastered the art and craft of the barber/surgeon you became *Master* of the guild, vulgarised to *Mister* over the centuries. A wonderful painting by Hans Holbein showing King Henry presenting the Royal Charter to Thomas Vickery, our first President, is on display in the great hall of the Royal College of Surgeons at Lincoln's Inn Fields to this day.

A few days later, whilst my balance of mind was still disturbed, and on my 28th birthday, I proposed marriage to Miss Judith Marcus on the town moor under the watchful eyes of the whitewall tyres of my doomed MGA. (Figure 12) To our surprise she accepted, but

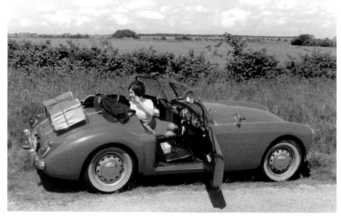

Fig. 12 Judy and my beloved MGA

which one of us she loved best at the time will never be known! I then approached her dad, Mr. Reuben Marcus, for permission to take his daughter's hand in marriage in a very formal and old-fashioned way. Ruby, as he was known, owned a tailoring business and was every inch a Geordie man: thick of accent, dour in countenance, wry in humour, a devotee of Newcastle United, and equally fond of his "Newcassel brun ale". Yet his grandparents grew up in a *stetl* in Eastern Europe as did my own. What chameleons we Jews are, my future father-in-law combining all the attributes of a Tyne-Tees man whilst retaining his orthodox Jewish allegiance. As far as he was concerned I was a suitable boy and we shook hands on the deal. My sweet little future mother-in-law Annie, who died with dignity at the age of 99 in 2006, was clearly overjoyed as by their ethnic standards her daughter, nearly 24, was already on the shelf.

We shared an engagement party in the hospital mess with Miles Irving and his lovely new fiancée Pat. (All four of us celebrated our ruby wedding anniversaries in 2005). Judy stunned my friends by turning up in a tight and dangerously short silk dress that heralded the era of the miniskirt and we jived to the music of the Mersey beat.

A few days later something terrible happened, an adumbration of a problem that would haunt me for decades to come – I experienced my first panic attack. I was seated at supper after a long day's work when suddenly I couldn't breathe. I experienced a sense of impending death. I thrashed around like a headless chicken to the consternation of my mess-mates. Eventually following a barbiturate sedative they got me to lie down in bed and sent for the duty physician. After a couple of days I was diagnosed with an acute anxiety/depressive illness brought on by overwork and loss of sleep and was prescribed anxiolytic drugs plus 10 days holiday. As chance would have it one of my best friends was getting married in Saudersfoot, South Wales, and I was invited to be an usher. So Judy, the MG and I went off for a few days relaxation, the first I had enjoyed in nearly a year. I remained haunted by the fear of another attack and noted prodromal symptoms whenever I was in a crowded and noisy place. However this was nothing like as bad as the horrors I experienced in 1984. (see chapter 11)

On September the 12th 1965 Judy and I were married in Leaze's Park synagogue next door to the football ground, with my youngest brother David, my best friend, acting as best man. (Figure 13) I have little memory of that event as I was drugged up to the eyebrows in

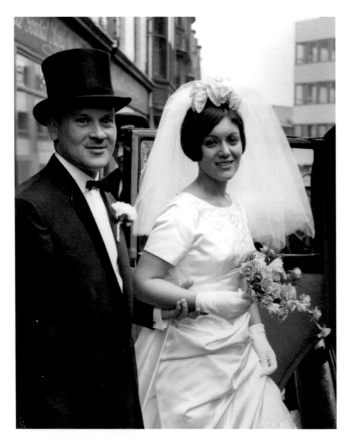

Fig. 13 Wedding picture

order to keep me standing still for 40 minutes under the *chupah* (Bridal canopy). Photographs of the event with my bride looking radiant and me looking bemused certainly confirm that the marriage took place and I have the *ketubah* (religious marriage contract) to prove it as well. We honeymooned in Ibiza before it became fashionable and shortly afterwards Mr. & Mrs. Baum travelled to London where I had been lucky enough to win a Cancer Research Campaign grant to study at King's College Hospital and Medical School in Denmark Hill. Thus we started our married life in Dulwich Village, a leafy suburb in southeast London surrounded by some of the poorest and most violent neighbourhoods in the country.

♥♥♥♥♥♥♥

On my first day as a clinical research fellow in the academic department of surgery, Professor Greig Murray greeted me: a twinkly eyed, rugged and handsome Scottish gentleman.

He was one of the Edinburgh School of clinical academics that populated most of the London chairs of surgery. This was partly because the Scots had a greater appreciation of medical science than the English and partly because of the attraction of a lucrative private practice in Harley Street that lured most prominent London surgeons away at a time when private practice was denied the senior academic staff. Just as an interesting aside, Greig Murray was only the second Professor of Surgery at King's College London, the first being the great Lord Lister, the founder of antisepsis in surgery. So great was his fame in the late 19th century that all the college surgeons, jealous of his private practice, vowed they would never have another surgeon with the title Professor. Never in my wildest dreams at that time did I imagine that I would be the third Professor of Surgery 15 years later. Greig Murray was a warm and kindly man who insisted I joined him for a wee dram of the finest malt whenever we met to discuss the progress of my research. Although gastroenterology was his subject and his knowledge of cancer research minimal, he always encouraged me and took delight in my progress.

My other mentor at the time was Mr. Colin Howe, the senior lecturer in the department.

Colin was the brother of Sir Geoffrey Howe who later went on to be Minister of Health and then Chancellor. Colin was married to the daughter of Lord Brock, the very man who had inducted me into the Royal College of Surgeons. At first I was terrified of Mr. Howe, who came over as a bruiser and a bully, but quickly I learnt that his manner was an affectation acquired during his time in the USA working for the great Dr. Zollinger in Boston. In fact Colin was a brilliant teacher who was adored by all the medical students. His main contribution to my success was the way he taught me to write and present scientific papers. Sadly my progress in the laboratory was slow and frustrating. I was investigating the then fashionable theory that there was a natural immune response to cancer mounted by the body itself. If we could only understand this and stimulate these natural mechanisms then we might have a treatment for the disease. I won't bore the reader with details but three decades of research in this area, all over the world, at huge expense, has lead nowhere. Certainly as far as breast cancer is concerned there is no such thing as immunotherapy. I remain wryly amused by the proponents of alternative therapy when they continually bang on about stimulating the immune system. They remind me of that stereotypical quack, Sir Ralph Bloomfield-Bonnington, in Shaw's "The Doctor's Dilemma", who believed that there was one sure cure for all disease, which was to "stimulate the phagocytes". My contribution to this subject was merely to increase the mortality of hundreds of inbred white mice in return for which I increased the volume of scientific "phenomenology". Since then I've had an aversion to animal studies, not because of any sentimental anthropomorphism but mainly because I soon learnt that the proper study of man was man (read woman) himself. However I made two exceptions to this principle, one I wish to explain now and the second later in this chapter.

One valuable aspect of this time as a research fellow was the freedom to read and think.

For example with the encouragement of my brother Harold I read scientific philosophy and became a devotee of Karl Popper (his name will crop up later). Next I became enthralled by the writings of Dr. Bernard Fisher of the University of Pittsburgh PA.

Throughout the 1960s Bernie Fisher was conducting a series of seminal experiments with *syngeneic* mice bearing transplantable tumours. Syngeneic means effectively that this strain of mice were all identical twins, therefore if one should develop a cancer you could transplant it to any of its litter mates without fear of rejection through the recently described mechanisms of *cell mediated immunity.* He therefore had an elegant experimental model that could at last challenge the dogma concerning the spread of cancer. The received wisdom at the time was that breast cancer spreads along the lymphatics to be arrested in the regional lymph glands that act as filter traps. (I will expand on this at length in the next chapter.) Suffice it to say that Fisher's experiments refuted that belief and demonstrated that murine (mouse) breast cancer spread via the bloodstream and could bypass the lymph glands with impunity. Furthermore, if anything, removal of these healthy glands seemed to impair the prognosis. In other words removing the tumour itself whilst leaving the glands intact meant the mice lived longer. Well that was good news for mice but, as Sir Michael Woodruff once put it, "it would still remain a problem to persuade the mice to come to the clinic!" Perhaps the most provocative and shocking interpretation of these experiments was the principle he developed known as "biological predeterminism". Fisher argued that if the cancer cells spread via the blood stream then by the time a tumour is discovered it has already had the chance to seed distant metastases (secondaries) and the extent of this dissemination was biologically rather than chronologically determined. Radical surgery therefore was "shutting the stable door after the horse had bolted".

After a year in the laboratory and the birth of my first child Richard, I returned to clinical practice with once again long hours and nights and weekends on call. Over the passage of three years I trained in gastrointestinal (GI) surgery, cardiothoracic and urological surgery, whilst nights and weekends I dealt with all the trauma and surgical emergencies that pitched up at our A & E department. During my time in GI surgery, a brilliant young consultant surgeon, Mr. John Dawson, heavily influenced me. He also provided mentorship and taught me by example how to handle human tissue with delicacy and respect. His speciality was hepatobiliary surgery and he also maintained a presence in the lab. Under his direction I carried out a series of elegant experiments using rats this time rather than mice. Not only are they bigger but they are meaner and when they bit your thumb they wouldn't let go. I would like to describe these experiments not because they are related in any way to breast cancer but because they beautifully illustrate scientific method and stand as an example of how animal research *can* save human lives. John Dawson was investigating the so-called "hepato-renal syndrome". This described the phenomenon of kidney failure following surgery on deeply jaundiced patients. John proposed the theory that the bile in the blood combined with transient hypoxia (lack of oxygen) poisoned the kidneys. He then designed the experiments and I executed them. We took two strains of rats, one with normal metabolism, the white Wistar rat, and the others who were congenitally jaundiced, the Gunn rat. These yellow creatures were born with the congenital absence of the enzyme *glucuronyl transferase*. (Please stay with me, it will become clear in a moment.) This enzyme is responsible for converting the pigment haemoglobin from effete red blood cells, into a soluble form of bile (bilirubin diglucuronide) that can be excreted via the liver and the bile ducts into the small bowel, providing the stools with their characteristic colour. In the absence of this enzyme the bilirubin hangs around in the blood and the rats turn yellow.

Patients with obstructive jaundice are yellow because the normal bile can't get into the gut because of a blockage, commonly due to gallstones or cancer of the pancreas.

In these experiments I took four groups of rats, two from the Wistar cages and two from the Gunn cages. One group of each strain had the bile duct tied off and all four had 30 minutes of transient hypoxia of the kidneys produced by a soft clamp across the renal pedicle. The only group of rats that went on to develop renal failure was the white ones with obstructive jaundice induced by ligating their bile duct. In other words it was the combination of renal hypoxia plus high levels of conjugated bile that poisoned the kidneys. From these experiments we figured out a way of maintaining a high urinary output and good oxygenation when operating on patients with obstructive jaundice, thus saving countless lives over the years. All credit to John Dawson, who died tragically young from hepatitis picked up from a patient he was operating on who happened to be a carrier of the hepatitis B virus; a terrible death from an occupational hazard of a front line soldier fighting to save human lives.

Thoracic surgery was something else. The way into the chest is more complicated than the way into the abdomen but when you get there the view is spectacular: all pink and shiny with the pleural lining of the chest cavity and covering the lungs reflecting the powerful operating lights. The lungs expanding and collapsing under the anaesthetist's control can be hypnotic as their marbled surface appears and disappears through the chest wall defect. All this in a patient of good health of course. Sadly in those cases operated upon for lung cancer the damage already suffered from years of tobacco abuse made the lungs look black, stiff and ugly. I soon became skilled at lobectomy and pneumonectomy for cancer, although it had its frightening moments. The low pressure high volume system of the right side of the heart means that any damage to the pulmonary veins causes the chest cavity to fill up with dark blood before you can identify the vascular defect. There was one exciting occasion when I was called to A & E to attend to a young man who had been stabbed in the right side of the chest in a pub brawl. He was rapidly exsanguinating so I rushed him to theatre, not sure if the blade had punctured his liver or lung. In fact the blade had "kebabed" the lung and entered the right ventricle, so he was effectively losing his life's blood in front of my eyes. I rapidly sewed up the defect with my assistant sucking out a couple of litres of blood and by some miracle he survived. A couple of days later whilst doing my ward round I was begged by the nursing staff to do something about this foul-mouthed stabee. Apparently he was effing and blinding at all the staff and making a bloody nuisance of himself. He cursed me when I raised the subject, so at visiting time I called his mother aside and explained the situation. Her response was enlightening and her very words were, "why don't you piss off". Ah well, that's the cultural norm for the badlands of South London I suppose.

This was the first cardiac operation I did alone and perhaps the last. Open-heart surgery with cardio-pulmonary by-pass was in its infancy and the consultants themselves were experiencing an unacceptable operative mortality so I remained a second assistant.

If the patient survived the operation I had to sleep next door to the intensive care unit (ICU) in case there was a crisis, whereas if the patient died on the table I went home to bed. I remember ringing Judy on a regular basis to tell her the good news that a patient survived and the bad news that I wouldn't be home until the following night.

In fact for the best part of the year I had no time off except for a Thursday evening.

However Thursdays were research days and a manic senior lecturer, Mr. Pat Cullum, was hoping to be the first to successfully carry out a heart transplant. For practice he and I used pigs. I anaesthetised the pig and inserted a very long laryngeal tube to keep the lungs inflated. The cardio-pulmonary technician (who incidentally ran the best fish and chip shop in Camberwell in his spare time!) put the pig on bypass. Pat and I then took out the heart, waited for half an hour and then sewed it back in. It seemed a pretty futile exercise to me at the time. Most of the pigs died so I could go home to bed but I remember our first success when I phoned up Judy with the good news that the pig had lived and the bad news that I would have to sleep with it all night whilst monitoring its vital signs every two hours. Pat Cullum and I nearly came to blows over this but eventually parted as good friends. Somewhere deep in my CV is a publication by Cullum and Baum describing the first successful porcine heart transplant.

Eventually after serving my apprenticeship in the sub specialities I was promoted to the position of lecturer and honorary senior registrar in the department of surgery. This is the equivalent of assistant professor or chief resident in the American system. It also marked the bifurcation in the pathway between a purely service position with consultancy in the NHS together with a lucrative private practice or the academic path that might lead to a chair in surgery with the denial of the right to private practice. As well as honing my skills in general surgery I started to take my teaching and research responsibilities very seriously. It was about this time that I decided to devote my career to the study of breast cancer.

The King's Cambridge trial

Perhaps the most important legacy of my time at King's as a lecturer in the department of surgery was the establishment of the first large multi-centre trial to study the treatment of breast cancer in the UK and I think at the time in Europe as a whole.

Working with a young research fellow in the department, Michael Edwards, (a kindly and thoughtful gentle-man who went on to enjoy a successful career loyally serving the NHS as a general surgeon), we developed an idea for a revolutionary trial that might challenge the conventional approach to the management of breast cancer. At the time we were heavily influenced by two groups of publications: firstly the work of Bernie Fisher and his mouse models, and secondly the studies on the "curability of breast cancer" by Dianna Brinkley and John Haybittle. Fisher's mouse studies suggested that if the regional lymph nodes (i.e. the glands draining the lymphatic tissue fluid from any anatomical region of the body) were not involved with cancer then that suggested an intact immune system mediated by those glands and therefore better left well alone. But if they were involved with cancer then that immune system was exhausted and the involvement of the nodes was the *expression* not the *determinant* of the poor prognosis. In other words if you removed normal glands you might impair outcome whereas the removal of involved glands was merely treating a symptom rather than curing the disease. A bit like trying to cure malaria by cooling the patient down during a crisis. Brinkley and Haybittle's work supported this concept by demonstrating unequivocally the "incurability" of breast cancer when treated by radical mastectomy. I will enlarge on this in the chapter on the natural history of breast cancer.

Suffice it to say that in following up a large series of women from the Cambridge data base, for more than 20 years, they were never able to define a point at which the mortality in the breast cancer group paralleled the mortality of age-matched women without breast cancer.

Emboldened by these findings with the rather cavalier attitude that there was nothing to lose, we designed a randomized controlled trial comparing a conventional approach of total mastectomy plus radiotherapy in place of surgery to control the disease in the axilla, versus surgery alone with *no* treatment of the axilla other than a watchful waiting policy that allowed delayed therapy if the swollen glands progressed sufficiently to become a clinical problem on their own. This was absolute heresy! In retrospect even if it was not heresy it was outrageous *chutzpah*. What was so surprising though was the incredible support the young Baum and Edwards received from our senior colleagues.

Professor Murray put his head on the block in our support. Mr. Brian Truscott, senior surgeon to Addenbrooke's hospital, joined the team. John Haybittle became our statistician and it was he who explained the importance of the large numbers needed to have the statistical "power" for discovering with confidence the modest but important differences in outcome. This is a statistical truism that I beg you to take on trust for the time being. He did the "power calculations" and concluded that we would need to recruit over 2,000 patients to be confident of finding a clinically important difference in outcome of about 7% in 10 year survival. Finally the glamorous and charming Dianna Brinkley joined us at King's as head of radiotherapy and added her name to the membership of the trial steering committee. Mike Edwards and I were then faced with the reality of recruiting 2,000 patients at a time when our own hospital treated about 150 cases a year. We packed our bags and filled cases with protocols and proformas and travelled round the UK covering different geographical areas. We even recruited centres in Copenhagen and Auckland, although how that came about I'm blowed if I can remember. Our host centres were generous with their time and we must have been persuasive with our arguments as we had no difficulty in recruiting enough centres, and in the fullness of time recruited more than 3,000 patients. The trial started in 1969 without the need for ethical approval or informed consent, something that haunts me to this day, but that was the *zeitgeist* of the period. It has to be remembered that we were pioneering the concept of multicentre collaboration, something upon which I've built my career, and we had no infrastructure to support this massive undertaking: just me and Mike and a secretary with a benevolent professor looking on. We made many mistakes and learnt quickly on the job. The worst error we made was in assuming that all our partners shared our beliefs about the scientific integrity of randomization. We learnt much later that a couple of centres would take the proffered brown envelope that held the randomized allocation, would then hold up the envelope to the theatre light, and if they didn't like what they saw take the next envelope in the bundle.

Although with the wisdom of hindsight the biological rationale of the study was naïve, the long term follow up of this group of patients provided valuable insights into the disease and its management that we never would have dreamed of. In my opinion Mike Edwards never enjoyed the credit he deserved for this massive undertaking. I will return to the long term results of this trial that revolutionized treatment in a way we never predicted in my chapter describing my years as professor of surgery at King's. However, before we get into that, I want to introduce my readers to the "natural history" and "unnatural history" of this tragic and enigmatic disease so that they may understand the fascination the subject had for me. I first describe the "unnatural" history of the cruel and futile attempts to cure breast cancer in the days before there was any understanding of normal human biology and physiology, never mind any understanding of the process of malignancy.

Chapter 5

The "Unnatural" History of Breast Cancer

Introduction

Each October is designated as breast cancer awareness month. This involves an intense campaign using billboards, leaflets and the sale of pink promotional ribbons and wristbands. The laudable objective of this campaign is to persuade women to be alert to changes in the texture or contour of their breasts that may indicate the early signs of breast cancer. It is then the unspoken assumption that if women "catch it early" they will save their breast and save their life. If only it was that simple! As the American humorist H.L. Menken once put it; "for every complex problem there is a simple solution and it's wrong". It is not the object of this book to dissuade women from being breast aware in the conventional sense but to open up the subject in such a way as to teach women, and for that matter men, about the extraordinary complexity of the disease, its extraordinary history and the extraordinary progress we have made in our understanding that has lead to the dramatic falls in breast cancer mortality in the United Kingdom, that have nothing to do with "catching it early". To achieve this understanding it is necessary for the lay person to join me first on a journey from the time of the Ancient Egyptians to the present in order to learn how false assumptions about the nature of breast cancer gave rise to cruel and futile interventions that added to the sum of human suffering. Next it is necessary to try and understand the "natural history" of the disease (i.e. what would happen if it was left to its own devices).

Finally it is also imperative to understand the exquisite mechanisms by which normal human tissue maintains its anatomical and functional integrity in order to understand what goes wrong during malignant transformation. Only with this understanding at the cell and molecular level can we start putting things right with rational biological approaches that have started paying dividends from the mid 1980s, leading me to believe that we are at a crossroads in the history of the subject. In order to make deaths from breast cancer a thing of the past we need the collaboration of the lay public to join in clinical trials and to keep faith with the scientific process, before the march of unreason extinguishes the illumination of the age of enlightenment. This is another of the reasons why I was provoked to write this book, not just to educate but also to warn that our hard-won advances are at risk by the flight from rational thinking.

Ancient Egypt (Figure 14)

A few years ago one of my brightest medical students joined my tutorial almost breathless with excitement, knowing my interest in breast cancer and the history of medicine. She had recently returned from an elective attachment in Egypt and had taken the opportunity of visiting the temples at Karnak. There she noted and photographed a low-relief statue of a woman who appeared to have only one breast. This find convinced her that the ancient Egyptian woman must have undergone a mastectomy for breast cancer. I do everything in my power to maintain the enthusiasm and powers of observation of my students but on this occasion, with much regret, I had to inform that she was wrong on two counts: first the history of art and second the history of medicine.

Pharaoh Djoser of the third dynasty (2686–2613 BCE), under the guidance of his chief minister, Imhotep, built the step pyramid at Sakkara with a neighbouring stone palace which for the first time in history included rows of pillars and walls decorated with low relief hieroglyphs. These low relief statues became encoded into a uniform and canonical style of such elegance that they continue to be rediscovered by fashionistas to this day. Imhotep was later revered as a God being credited with life saving advances in medicine as well as art and architecture and was later conflated with the Greek god of healing, Asclepius. So the idea of doctors playing God is not new either.

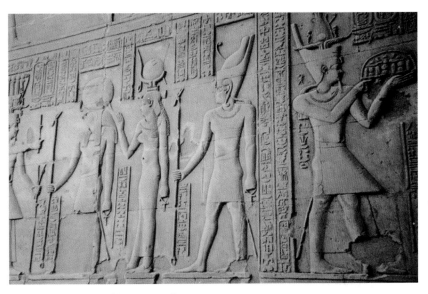

Fig. 14 Temple wall at Karnak

The canonical style for the depiction of men, women and gods was strictly defined. Men were shown with the trunk facing the observer and their legs in profile whereas women were shown in perfect profile along the full length of their bodies (although their lower limbs were often covered in see-through pleated muslin that is still seductive to the eye). Pharaohs and gods were seen with head, trunk and lower legs in a full frontal pose either sitting or striding purposefully towards the observer. As women were shown only in stylised profile then the breasts are superimposed one upon the other giving a misleading appearance.

However of greater interest to this subject we actually have documentary evidence that the ancient Egyptians recognised breast cancer but specifically counselled against mastectomy! (Figure 15)

"If thou examinest a man/woman having bulging tumours of his/ her breast and thou findest that the swellings have spread over his/her breast; if thou puttest your hand upon his/her breast upon these tumours, and thou findest them very cool, there being no fever at all herein when thy hand touches him/her; they have no granulations, they form no fluid, they do not generate secretions of fluid and they are bulging to thy hand. Thou should say concerning him/her, there is no treatment".

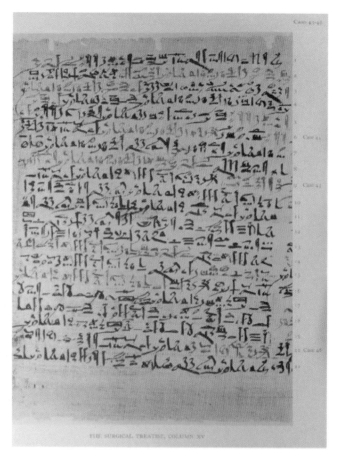

Fig. 15 Edwin Smith papyrus

This translation of the Edwin Smith surgical papyrus (3000BCE-2500BCE), by J.H. Breasted was published in 1930 and the papyrus itself can be seen in the Chicago Institute of Art. Is this the first example of breast cancer awareness?

Many scholars have suggested that the ancient Egyptians are here distinguishing breast cancer from inflammatory mastitis. I would go further and suggest that having excluded inflammation, lactational mastitis and cysts, the ancient Egyptian has defined a new class of disease that only gets worse with surgical interference. As the swelling described has spread over the breast then he must be describing locally advanced breast cancer. We have learnt to our cost that in this stage of the disease surgery makes things worse. The wisdom of this ancient was lost for over 4000 years as generations of surgeons and physicians made futile attempts to cure advanced breast cancer with unimaginably cruel consequences. Apart from describing breast cancer this papyrus was perhaps the first expression of the old medical maxim, "there are many conditions that you cannot help but there are none you cannot make worse".

Around 400 BCE, Hippocrates, the great grandfather of modern medicine, went even further when he wrote 'It is better to give no treatment in cases of hidden cancer (referring to non-ulcerating breast cancer); treatment causes speedy death, but to omit treatment is to prolong life'. *"primum non nocere".*

Hippocrates went on to develop his ideas concerning the natural humours of the body and to suggest that cancer like most other disease processes resulted from an imbalance of these humours, but as far as I can judge he never described how these humoural imbalances could be corrected to the advantage of patients with breast cancer. Perhaps at this point a short digression is necessary to explain the concept of the "natural humours" promoted by Aristotle and Hippocrates that were central to medical beliefs right up until the early 19thC and are enjoying a return to fashion as "ancient wisdom" in the promotion of alternative medicine. Central to the Hippocratic teachings was the belief that health was a state of equilibrium and sickness the result of an imbalance. What were being kept in balance were bodily fluids or "humours". These fluids were in part real and in part metaphysical. The fluids that we can recognize today are blood, yellow bile and phlegm but the fourth,"black bile", has no modern equivalent. These humours were linked to the four elements (blood/air, yellow bile/fire, black bile/earth, phlegm/water) and to the personality of the patient using descriptive terms that are still in use; "sanguine", "choleric", "melancholic" and "phlegmatic". Blood made the body hot and wet e.g. fever, choler made the body hot and dry e.g. eczema, phlegm cold and wet e.g. tuberculosis and black bile cold and dry e.g. cancer. Diagnosis for the balance of the humours was made by examining the urine held up to the light and by noting the volume of the pulse.

This scheme finds parallels in traditional Chinese and Indian medicine. It is interesting to note that women with breast cancer were said to be of a melancholic type because they were often depressed – another condition claimed to be due to an excess of black bile. Of course this was an early example of confusion in the direction of causality. In other words depression doesn't cause breast cancer but the disease can make women depressed!

In the absence of any useful therapy on offer women sought spiritual solace and miraculous healing with prayer and votive offerings at the temples of Asclepius. A votive offering to the gods is usually in the form of a model of the diseased part of the body. A beautiful example of a marble votive offering can be seen in the Louvre gallery in Paris (Figure 16) although to my eyes the right breast shows the signs of a giant benign fibroadenoma rather than a cancer.

A few years ago I was at a meeting in Naples hosted by my friend Professor Rafelle Bianco, a distinguished medical oncologist. Once the meeting was over he took me on a sightseeing trip to hidden parts of the city. The city was founded by refugees from the Greek mainland in about 500 BCE and was originally called Neapolis (new city). Deep underground in the old centre of the city there are remarkable excavations where you can trace the history of Naples through various strata built one upon the other. The deepest layer is from the times of the ancient Greeks and there you will see the remains of a temple devoted to Asclepius. Above that you can visit

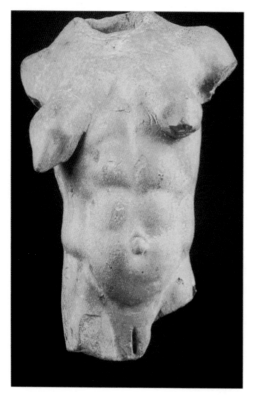

Fig. 16 Marble torso as votive offering, The Louvre

the remains of a Roman temple. One more layer of history brings you to a Byzantine church. Finally superimposed on these footprints of the spiritual history of Naples you enter the Roman Catholic Church of San Lorenzo built about 150 years ago. Professor Bianco took me into a side chapel there and showed me walls covered with votive offerings including countless metallic plaques with low relief images of the breast. I asked him when this practice ended. Without a word he guided me to the local market and bought me a gift of such a votive offering. (Figure 17) The hairs on the nape of my neck bristled as I envisaged 2000 years of women suffering from breast cancer attending this divine spot, praying to their gods, seeking a miraculous cure or at least spiritual solace. We should resist mocking these superstitions and constantly remind ourselves of the need we all feel for the transcendental when facing existential threats.

Approximately 500 years after Hippocrates, during the flowering of the Greco/Roman period of medicine, Celsus made probably the first attempt to describe, classify and stage carcinoma of the breast. He suggested four stages, (1) Early malignancy (2) Cancer without ulcer (3) Ulcerating cancer and (4) Fungating (literally looking like a fungus) cancer. In contrast to the teachings of Hippocrates he felt that treatment, although contraindicated in the three late stages, might be of some value in the earliest stage. Although what treatment he had in mind remains obscure. In approximately 200 AD, Galen, who studied

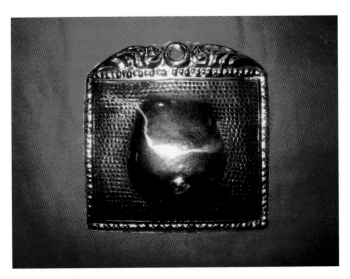

Fig. 17 Modern day votive offering Naples

in Alexandria and practiced in Rome, became the most influential physician of the then known world. He further extended the Hippocratic humoural theory of disease and taught that cancer was related to the accumulation of an excess of black bile (melancholia) that coagulated in the breast. He supported this view by suggesting that women clear themselves of black bile during their monthly periods and therefore after the menopause they are no longer cleansed. This conveniently explained the increasing incidence of breast cancer amongst women in their fifth and sixth decades. If such was the case it would appear logical to cleanse the women again by repeated purgation and bleeding, coupled with diets with a low capacity of producing black bile. These approaches were also used for the treating of depression as described in Alan Bennett's wonderful play "The Madness of King George", and are enjoying something of a renaissance with the Gerson regimen for cancer, an alternative remedy promoted by members of today's royal family. This is probably the first and one of the finest examples of what I like to describe as conceptual rationalizations of therapy for breast cancer. Note also that the disease was considered a systemic disorder, but that didn't stop physicians and proto-surgeons from using topical applications for ulcers and breast amputation for the smaller tumours. It is darkly comic to read how those ancient surgeons hazarding amputation of the breast were encouraged not to stop the bleeding too quickly in order to allow the excess of evil humours to escape. (Figure 18)

It is also a salutary lesson to remember that during the dark ages, amputation of the breasts was used as torture or as a method of execution, for female heretics. The most famous of these was St. Agatha, the patron saint of the breast. Agatha was born in Palermo, Sicily c. 250 CE. Young, beautiful and rich, Agatha lived a life consecrated to God. When the Roman Emperor Decius announced the edicts against Christians, the local magistrate Quintianus tried to profit by Agatha's sanctity – he planned to blackmail her into sex in exchange for not charging her. Handed over to a brothel, she refused to accept customers. After rejecting Quintianus' advances, she was beaten, imprisoned, tortured, her breasts were crushed and cut off. She told the judge, "Cruel man, have you forgotten your mother and the breast that nourished you, that you dare to mutilate me this way?" Legend has it that Saint Peter healed her before she eventually died by being rolled in burning coals.

The martyrdom of St. Agatha has been a popular subject for painters throughout the middle ages. I have seen many gruesome images of

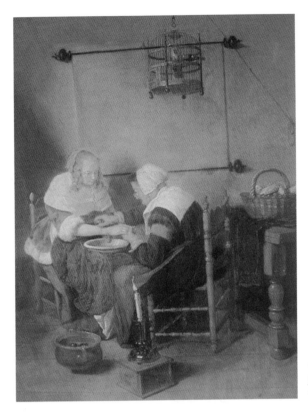

Fig. 18 Dutch genre painting of the leech woman

the event but my favourite, if you'll forgive the expression, is the painting by the Venetian artist, Jean Baptiste Tiepolo, completed in about 1750. (Figure 19)

You will note that the attendant on her left holds a bloody cloth to her chest, whilst her torturer triumphantly brandishes his blood stained sword. The attendant to Agatha's right holds a platter upon which rests her two neatly amputated breasts. Many of these depictions were misinterpreted and thought to show pastries with a cherry on top on the platter.!! For that reason Agatha has also become the patron saint of pastry cooks and on her saints day, 5th February, little cakes with cherries on top known as "mammilles santa Agatha", are traditionally served in many Catholic European countries.

Such was the charisma of Galen and so rapidly did his teachings become the orthodoxy that for almost 1200 years no one dared challenge his doctrine. The dark ages must have been very dark indeed for women with breast cancer, apart from the two fortunates who

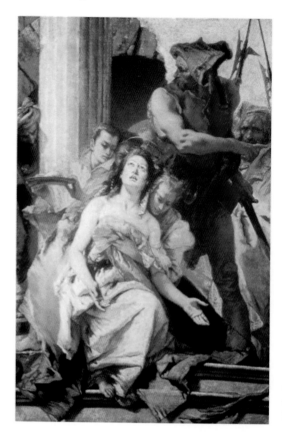

Fig. 19 The martyrdom of Saint Agatha, Jean Baptiste Tiepolo 1750

enjoyed miraculous cures of their disease through the ministrations of Saints Kosmas and Damian (The Patron Saints of the Royal College of Surgeons of England).

The Renaissance

The Renaissance is usually remembered as the rebirth of interest in the arts and culture of ancient Greece; with painting, sculpture and literature throwing off the shackles of the orthodox Catholic Church, the broadening of study to include liberal subjects and the precious gift of enquiry. This new found freedom of enquiry encouraged developments in anatomy and pathology but at the same time lead to some bizarre and infertile pathways in the treatment of cancer. For example, Ambrose Paré (1510–1590) the great French military surgeon, advised women against gossip in order to avoid breast cancer (perhaps also a great pre-Chauvin male chauvinist pig?) and recommended treating ulcerated cancer with puppy dogs or kittens freshly split into two with the warm viscera applied to the lesion. However, to his credit he did recognize that swelling of the lymph glands (axillary lymph nodes) in the armpit draining the cancer was a bad sign in the disease and advocated the use of ligatures to staunch the bleeding after surgery to remove the breast instead of the red hot irons. Wilhelm Fabry (1565–1634) also known as Fabricius, who practiced in Germany, considered that cancer was caused by milk curdling in the breast and is thought to have performed the first axillary node dissection via a counter incision in the armpit. (Mastectomy in those days was a simple guillotine amputation with cautery to control the haemorrhage. (Figure 20)

Gabriele Falloppio (1523–62) who was professor of anatomy and surgery at Padua, modified Galen's humoural theory and introduced a non-natural bile which was a combustion product of other humours.

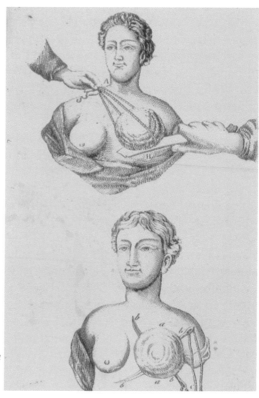

Fig. 20 Textbook illustration of a mastectomy from mid 18th C

He suggested that cancers consisted of a blend of blood and "burnt" melancholic humour with the degree of malignancy related to the relative proportions of these two substances, with inflammatory carcinoma having the worst prognosis as a result of the most disadvantageous combination. He was the first to describe fixation of the tumour to the underlying pectoral muscles of advanced breast cancer and used this physical sign as evidence of inoperability. Unfortunately he persisted in advising blood letting (venesection) to rid the body of burnt black bile (same treatment, different rationale!).

The 17th and 18th centuries

The start of the 17th century saw the beginning of the waning influence of the humoural theory of cancer in favour of particular theories of disease due to mechanical defects or hydrodynamic processes. These attitudes were no doubt brought about by Harvey's description of the circulation of the blood in 1628, together with the adoption of the Cartesian view of the body as a perfect machine. Thomas Bartholin (1616–1680) first described the lymphatic system allowing both humoural and mechanical theories of cancer to coexist. The tumours, it was suggested, were clotted tissue fluid (lymph) due to blockage of lymphatic vessels. But perhaps the most important development of this period that would in time allow a revolutionary approach to the understanding of cancer was the description of the first microscope by Antonie van Leeuwenhoek (1632–1723). This is but one example in the history of science where the invention of an instrument that extended the human powers of observation also extended the human capacity for the generation of hypotheses.

At the same time physicians were also arguing about the psychological trauma and contagious inductions of cancer, whilst still not capable of understanding how the patients died of secondary spread (metastases). For example, Nicholaes Tulp (1593–1674), the famous Dutch anatomist and surgeon, believed that patients died from autointoxication from their ulcerated cancers. He was also responsible for the single anecdote that convinced generations of doctors that breast cancer was a contagious disease, as a result of being called to treat both mistress and servant of the same household for cancer of the breast. Tulp was of course immortalized in Rembrandt's painting of 'The Anatomy Lesson'. (Figure 21) The artist himself unwittingly contributed to the subject in his hauntingly beautiful painting entitled 'Bathsheba at her toilet.' (Figure 22) As mentioned in an earlier

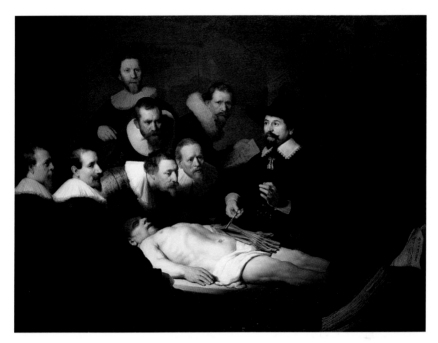

Fig. 21 The anatomy lesson of Nicholaes Tulp, by Rembrandt

chapter, the model for this work completed in 1655 was Rembrandt's mistress Hendrickje Stoffles. Careful examination of the upper outer quadrant of her left breast demonstrates the characteristic dimple of a cancer. She died 9 years after this painting was completed and her mode of dying was suggestive of metastatic breast cancer.

In the early 18th century tumours of all sorts were still grouped together with persistence of the ancient distinction between 'scirrhous' and 'carcinomatous' growths. The former were thought to be premalignant and the latter lethally malignant. The aetiology of the disease was still considered a combination of local and general (systemic) causes. The local causes included trauma, tight clothes and curdled milk, whilst the systemic factors were related to blood components, for example 'yellow bile' from serum; 'phlegm' from stagnant serum; 'black bile', the clot of extruded red blood cells; 'materia phlogistica' the component of blood thought to develop into pus. Most physicians favoured the theory that "materia phlogistica" coagulated internally to produce a scirrhous, although John Hunter (1728–1793) the influential London surgeon favoured the coagulated lymph theory. John Hunter, considered to be the father of British surgical science,

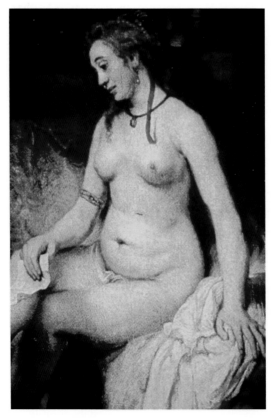

Fig. 22 Bathsheba at her toilet by Rembrandt

lived in a fashionable town house in Leicester Square. The gentry gained entry via the square whilst the grave robbers who supplied the cadavers for anatomical dissection gained access via a secret entrance in the mews round the back. Anyone who wishes to gain some insight into this turbulent period in the history of British surgery would be well advised to visit the Hunterian Museum at the Royal College of Surgeons, Lincoln's Inn Fields. Entrance is free to the lay public though I would advise you go before not after a heavy lunch!

Other theories abounded including ingestion of poisons, excess of acidity or alkalinity in the blood, psychological trauma, bad diet and failure to bear children (nulliparity). Nulliparity is recognised as a risk factor to this day and was first described by Ambrose Paré who noted a high incidence of the disease amongst the nuns in a convent he attended.

Perhaps the two most important conceptual advances of this period can be attributed to the French surgeons Le Dran (1685–1770) and

Petit (1674–1750) who explained the nature of metastases as either blood born (haematogenous) or lymphatic spread of the disease to the armpit (axilla) and distant organs. Unfortunately treatment was still lagging far behind conceptual advances with guillotine amputation in rare selected cases of early disease and disgusting topical applications, diet, purgation and bleeding for most other cases. However, for the first time we can see the adumbration of the controversy of conservative versus radical surgery that was to dominate the debate in the mid 20thC when William Cheseldon of St. George's Hospital London (1688–1752) started advocating just the removal of the malignant lump (lumpectomy) whilst Louis Petit of Paris was advocating the more radical approach with a total mastectomy. Ironically the London/Paris position became reversed in the mid 20thC.

The first reported long term survivor of mastectomy was a nun working as a nurse at L'Hôtel-Dieu, Quebec. The great Canadian surgeon Michel Sarrazin described her first visit to him in Montreal: *"Dès le petit printemps de l'année 1700, la chère sœur Marie Barbier de l'Assomption, Congréganiste, descendit de Montréal pour se faire guérir chez nous d'un cancer qu'elle avait au sein."*

He then goes on to describe her incredible fortitude under the surgeon's knife as she offered up her life to the service of God should she survive. She lived for 30 years and ended up as a much venerated mother superior of her convent.

The 19th century

Perhaps there is no better way of entering the 19thC than by quoting from the diary of Fanny Burney (Figure 23), a noted authoress and diarist of that time, with an entry from the year 1811:

"I mounted the bed stead, he placed me upon the mattress and spread a cambric handkerchief upon my face. It was transparent however and I saw through it, that the bed stead was instantly surrounded by seven men and my nurse. Through the cambric I saw the hand held up while his forefinger first described a straight line from top to bottom of the heart, secondly a cross and thirdly a circle; intimating that the whole was to be taken off.

When the dreadful steel was plunged into the heart cutting through veins-arteries-nerves, I needed no injunctions not to restrain my cries. I began a scream that lasted during the

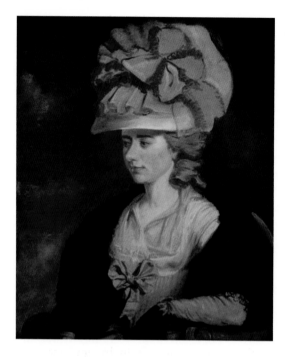

Fig. 23 Portrait of Fanny Burney, National Portrait Gallery

whole time of the incision and marvel that it rings not in my ears still.

When the wound was made and the instrument withdrawn the pain seemed undiminished, for the air that suddenly rushed into those delicate parts felt like sharp and forked poniards that were tearing the edges of the wound.

Again I felt the instrument describing a curve cutting against the grain, while the flesh resisted in a manner so forcible to oppose and tire the hand of the operator. I concluded the operation over – Oh No! The terrible cutting was renewed and worse than ever. I felt the knife crackling against the breast bone – scraping it! To conclude, the evil was so profound that the operation lasted twenty minutes."

Thus was the experience of a mastectomy before the days of anaesthetics, so it can easily be understood that the majority of women kept away from surgeons and favoured folk remedies.

"The Cook and Housekeeper's Complete and Universal Dictionary" compiled by Mrs. Mary Eaton at the beginning of the 19th century describes the popular management of cancer, slotted in alphabetical order between canaries and candied angelica. Mrs. Eaton suggested that – 'this cruel disorder" could be cured in 3 days by a simple application without the need of surgery. The topical agent was made from dough mixed with hog's lard applied to the affected part spread on a piece of white leather. She concludes – "This, if it do no good is perfectly harmless, several persons have derived great benefit from this application and it has seldom been known to fail'.

At the same time the medical establishment were asking themselves some very pertinent questions about the nature of cancer. In 1802 a meeting took place in Edinburgh at which were John Abernethy, John Hunter's pupil and his successor as Surgeon at St. Bartholomew's Hospital, Mathew Baillie a nephew of Hunter's and the author of 'Morbid Anatomy', Robert Willen, founder of dermatology, and John Hunter's brother-in-law, Everand. This committee discussed the question 'May cancer be regarded at any period or under any circumstances merely as a local disease, or does the existence of it in one part afford a presumption that there is a tendency to a familiar alteration in other parts of the animal?' The result of their deliberations was published in July 1806 in the Edinburgh Medical and Surgical Journal and to some extent pre-empted the debate that started in the 1950s. Nevertheless, breast cancer was by now assumed to be a localized disease requiring radical extirpation if cure was to be attempted. A beautiful and heartbreaking description of James Syme (Professor of Surgery in Glasgow and Lord Lister's father-in-law) performing a mastectomy in 1830, appears in the story 'Rab and his friends' by John Brown.

"The operating theatre is crowded; much talk and fun, and all the cordiality and stir of youth. The surgeon with his staff of assistants is there. In comes Ailie: one look at her quiets and abates the eager students. That beautiful old woman is too much for them; they sit down, and are dumb, and gaze at her. These rough boys feel the power of her presence. She walks in quickly, but without haste; dressed in her mutch, her neckerchief, her white dimity short-gown, her black bombazine petticoat, showing her white worsted stockings and her carpet shoes. Behind her was James with Rab. James sat down in the distance, and took that huge and noble head between his knees. Rab looked perplexed and dangerous; forever cocking his ear and dropping it as fast. Ailie stepped up on a seat, and laid herself on the table, as her friend the surgeon told her; arranged herself, gave a rapid

*look at James, shut her eyes, rested herself on me, and took
my hand. The operation was at once begun; it was necessarily
slow; and chloroform – one of God's best gifts to his suffering
children – was then unknown. The surgeon did his work. The
pale face showed its pain, but was still and silent. Rab's soul
was working within him; he saw that something strange was
going on, – blood flowing from his mistress, and she suffering;
his ragged ear was up, and importunate; he growled and gave
now and then a sharp impatient yelp; he would have liked to
have done something to that man. But James had him firm, and
gave him a glower from time to time, and an intimation of a
possible kick; – all the better for James, it kept his eye and
his mind off Ailie. It is over: she is dressed, steps gently and
decently down from the table, looks for James; then, turning to
the surgeon and the students, she courtesies, and in a low, clear
voice begs their pardon if she has behaved ill. The students – all
of us – wept like children; the surgeon clapped."*

The courageous woman survived this procedure only to die of
septicaemia in the following week. James Syme could hardly be
blamed for this in the era before Lister's revolutionary discoveries lead
to the development of antiseptic techniques. Syme is to be credited
as the first to make the association between involved axillary nodes
and the systemic nature of the disease. In 1842 he wrote as follows:
'The result of operations for carcinoma when the glands are affected
is almost always unsatisfactory however perfectly they may seem to
have been taken away. The reason for this is probably that the glands
do not take part in the disease unless the system is strongly disposed
to it'. I will return to this important insight in the next chapter.

Improvements in the microscope in the mid 19th century allowed
the study of the cellular aspects of cancer and the foundation of cancer
histology as a science. This science was held back by problems with
the interpretation of artefacts due to the poor preparation of specimens.
It is likely that these artefacts led to the 'Blastema' theory of cancer
promoted by Karl Rokitansky (1804–1878) and Sir James Paget (1814–
1899). The 'Blastema' was considered to be a primitive form of cell
seen as a solid amorphous substance under the microscope, capable
of giving rise to cancers at any site within the supporting structures
of healthy organs. This view was attacked by Rudolf Virchow (1821–
1902) who suggested that cancers arose from normal cells in reaction
to abnormal stimuli, a singularly modern viewpoint. Yet paradoxically

it was Virchow who promoted the view of the centrifugal spread of cancer along the lymphatics by cellular migration whilst Sir James Paget believed in a humoural mechanism of metastasis via the blood stream. Virchow's viewpoint became dominant and contributed to the evolution of the radical mastectomy. (*vide infra*)

The late 19th century and early 20th century

The late 19th century marked the transformation of surgery by the twin developments of anaesthesia and antisepsis.

In 1867, twenty years after the first anaesthetic (ether) was given by Dr. William Thomas Green Morton in Boston, Massachusetts, a forty-four year-old Londoner called Isabella Pim discovered a large lump growing in her breast. She first went to see Sir James Paget of Wimpole Street, but he explained that the dangers of surgery were too great, because the cancer was at an advanced stage. Unwilling to accept this advice, she travelled to Edinburgh to see James Syme, her brother's father-in-law, for a second opinion. He also advised that the risks of surgery outweighed the benefits.

Finally she went to her brother, Joseph Lister, the Professor of Surgery at the Glasgow Royal Infirmary. Shortly before her visit he had published a series of articles in *The Lancet* that would revolutionize the practice of surgery. In them he had described how he had improved the chances of survival for patients with compound fractures of the bone (that is fractures where the sharp ends of the broken bone had punctured the skin). Whilst previously, about half of such patients would die of hospital diseases, ten out of eleven of Lister's survived.

Lister's breakthrough was dependent on a new understanding of the mechanism of infection. Two years previously, he had read the publications of Louis Pasteur that laid the groundwork for the bacterial theory of post-operative infection. Lister applied these principles to prevent infection in the operating theatre resulting from bacterial contamination in the air, on the clothes of the surgeon and on the surgical instruments that were usually covered in a patina of blood and fat from previous patients on the operating room list. A dilute solution of carbolic acid was to be sprayed in the air of the operating theatre, soaked into the lint of dressings and used to clean the scalpel and forceps. (Figure 24) When his sister sought his advice, the method had so far only been used to treat abscesses and compound fractures. One can easily imagine Lister's torment. Although he was convinced

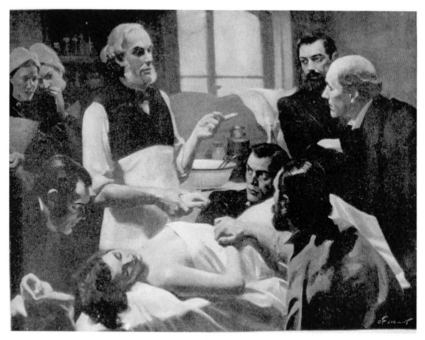

Fig. 24 Lord Lister in operating theatre

of his own method, most other surgeons were deeply sceptical. What if his sister would die under his knife? How could he then live with his conscience and what would that do for the future of his experimental technique? So he too travelled to Edinburgh to consult his father-in-law and mentor James Syme who gave him the courage to proceed.

Although Lister had done a number of mastectomies, he took the precaution of practising the operation on a cadaver. Shortly before the operation he wrote to his father as follows; 'I suppose before this reaches thee the operation of darling Bella will be over. It is very satisfactory to me that B seems to have thorough confidence in me. She distinctly says she would much rather have me to perform the operation than anyone else. And considering *what* the operation is to be I would rather not let anyone else do it.' On the day following the operation he again wrote to his father; 'I may say that the operation was at least as well as if she had not been my sister. But I do not wish to do such a thing again.' In the days that followed, the wound did not turn septic. (At this point I must empathise with Lister. 120 years after this event my own sister consulted me with her breast cancer but fortunately unlike Lister I had countless others I could trust with my sister's life.)

Seven weeks after the operation, Lister went to Dublin to present a paper at a British Medical Association meeting. Whereas previously he had advocated his technique for fractures and abscesses, now he presented it as a general method 'On the Antiseptic Principle in the Practice of Surgery'. Since he had started using it himself, he declared, not a single case of hospital gangrene had appeared on his wards. Surprisingly Lister's techniques were slow to catch on amongst the ultra conservative medical establishment in the UK. He became very frustrated with the way he was treated by his peers in Scotland and readily accepted the position as the first Professor of Surgery at King's College Hospital London. From this base his fame and private practice burgeoned, hospital mortality plummeted and he was elevated to the House of Lords. The statue of Lord Lister, the only one of a surgeon in the capital, can be seen on Portland Place, just round the corner from where I work at the Portland Hospital. The other thing we have in common is that I became the third Professor of Surgery at King's College. The second, Greig Murray, another Scot, was appointed about 60 years after Lister's death. The long hiatus was due to the jealousy felt by the Harley Street mafia at the large private practice Lister attracted, who vowed that the title gave its bearer an unfair advantage in the market place in the days leading up to the establishment of the NHS.

With the developments of anaesthesia and antisepsis surgeons were at last released from their shackles, and providing blood loss was adequately controlled almost anything outside the chest and skull was possible. Of course whether it was desirable was another question!

The development of the classical radical mastectomy in the latter part of the nineteenth century is usually credited to William S. Halsted, of the Johns Hopkins Hospital, Baltimore (1898). (Figure 25) But it has to be remembered that the operation was designed on the basis of the pathological teachings of Virchow described above. It was assumed that a cancer spread in continuity from its origin as columns of malignant cells. These passed along the lymphatic channels until they were arrested temporarily in the first group of regional lymph nodes, which were thought to act as filter traps. It was further assumed that when the filtration capacity of these lymph nodes was exhausted they acted as a nidus for tertiary spread to more distant lymph nodes and then via the tissue planes to the skeleton and the vital organs. Halsted even went so far as to suggest that

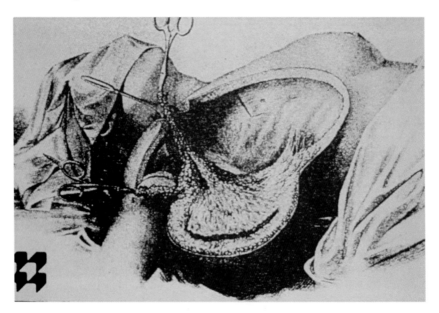

Fig. 25 Classical Halsted radical mastectomy

there was no skeletal involvement unless there was an overlying skin secondary with the skeleton being involved as a result of continuity from the original growth via the skin metastasis. Accepting these beliefs it seemed quite reasonable that radical surgery that included all the lymph channels and their nodes/glands in the axilla would cure more patients than local amputation of the breast alone. Furthermore it stood to reason that the operation had to be completed *en bloc* in order to prevent the spillage of cancer cells into the wound by cutting across lymphatic channels. For a short period in the early 1920s some surgeons were taking this matter to the logical conclusion and advocating amputation of the arm at the shoulder together with radical clearance of the breast when the disease had spread locally into the upper arm. For that matter, it must be remembered that in the mid 20thC the super-radical mastectomy was advocated that included lifting up the sternum like a trap door and dissecting out the lymph glands that ran down the front of the chest cavity.

In 1898 Marie Curie discovered the extraordinary properties of the unstable element, radium. She was awarded the Nobel Prize for this discovery in 1911. By that time a primitive form of radiotherapy was already in use for the treatment of breast cancer. The remarkable painting of Dr. Chicotot delivering radiation to the breast can be seen in Paris at the Musée de L'assistance Publique. It was completed in 1907 and the artist was the good doctor himself. (Figure 26)

I note with wry amusement the long white apron and top hat. The former was not just for hygiene but to this day is considered a badge of office for senior physicians who have earned their post-graduate doctorate. Unfortunately the starched linen did little to protect the gonads of the doctor from scattered radiation, unlike the lead apron of later years. Sadly many of these pioneers, including Marie Curie herself, died of cancer induced by radiation; a double-edged weapon indeed. I once had the rare privilege of visiting Madame Curie's original laboratory at the Institute Curie in Paris: visitors are few and far between and only allowed 20 minutes at the maximum. I was shown the star exhibit – her notebook describing the physical properties of radium. My guide held a Geiger counter over the glass case and it went crazy. I leapt back in alarm and exited well before my 20 minutes were up.

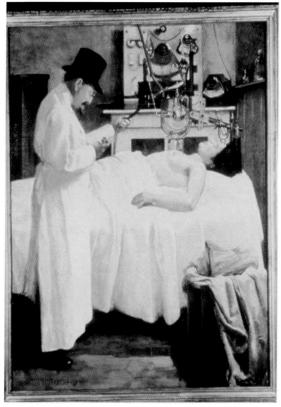

Fig. 26 Dr. Chicotot

The research of Marie Curie was to have a lasting effect on the management of breast cancer.

In 1922 Geoffrey Keynes, surgeon at St. Bartholomew's Hospital London, began experimenting with the use of radium enclosed in hollow platinum needles in the treatment of advanced breast cancer. (Figures 27, 28) Keynes, later Sir Geoffrey, was a remarkable man born from the most remarkable genetic pool in the United Kingdom. His genealogy included the blood of the Darwins, Wedgwoods and Huxleys. He was the brother of the great economist Maynard Keynes, and grew up in a hot house of culture and intellectual enquiry. In addition to being a great and innovative surgeon he was also a collector of the works of the 18thC visionary poet and painter William Blake. In fact after his retirement he enjoyed a second career as an art historian and completed the bibliography of Blake and his followers.

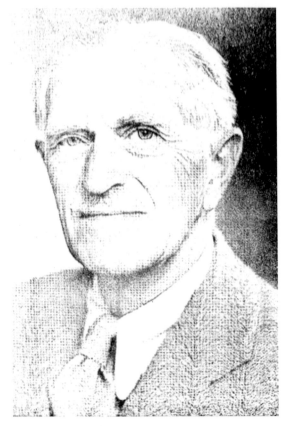

Fig. 27 Sir Geoffrey Keynes

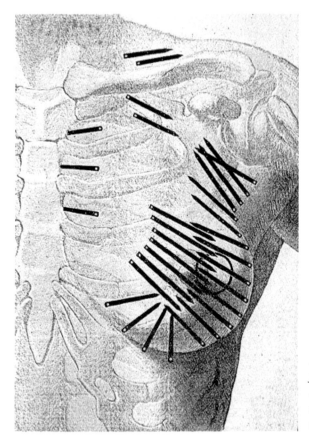

Fig. 28 Illustration from the BMJ 1935 showing Keynes' approach to breast conserving surgery

All this can be read in his wonderful autobiography, "The Gates of Memory", published in his 94th year.

Following on from his experience with advanced disease he then took the courageous leap of faith and started treating women with early breast cancer with local excision (lumpectomy) and radium needles inserted into the unaffected quadrants of the breast and the axillary plus supra-clavicular lymphatic fields. This was considered heresy at the time yet his results at ten year follow-up published in the BMJ in 1936 looked as good as anything that the radical mastectomy had to offer. Unfortunately before he had a chance to popularize his technique the Second World War broke out and Sir Geoffrey was called to serve his country as senior surgeon to the RAF. For safety sake his radium needles were buried safely deep underground and with that his technique was buried, only to be resurrected some twenty years after VE day.

There is a curious and sinister story, which just might be true, linking breast cancer to the outbreak of WWII. Here I acknowledge the plagiarism from an extraordinary blog; http://scienceblogs.com/ insolence/2006/04/mrs_hitler_and_her_doctor.php

****

In 1907, Adolf Hitler's mother Klara died of breast cancer at age 47, when Hitler was only 18. The young Hitler was devastated by her death. Indeed, in *Mein Kampf*, Hitler described her death as follows:

> *These were the happiest days of my life and seemed to me almost a dream; and a mere dream it was to remain. Two years later, the death of my mother put a sudden end to all my highflown plans.*
>
> *It was the conclusion of a long and painful illness which from the beginning left little hope of recovery. Yet it was a dreadful blow, particularly for me. I had honored my father, but my mother I had loved.*

Dr. Eduard Bloch, the family physician who diagnosed and treated Klara Hitler's breast cancer was, through an odd quirk of fate, Jewish. Consequently it is not surprising that some, such as Rudolf Binion, have speculated that a hatred of Dr. Bloch for "failing" to save his mother might have been one factor behind Hitler's later violent anti-Semitism and even may have resulted in the Holocaust. It is argued, contrary to the criticisms that were later leveled against Bloch, that Dr. Bloch actually performed his treatments competently according to the prevailing medical standards of the time. Sandy MacCleod an Australian psychologist and historian, describes Klara's initial presentation as follows:

> *Mrs Hitler saw Dr Bloch on 14 January 1907 complaining of a chest pain, 'so severe it interrupted sleep'. She was described by her doctor as 'a simple, modest, kindly woman, tall with brownish hair which she kept neatly plaited, and a long oval face with beautifully expressive grey-blue eyes'. Quiet, pious and maternal, three of her children had died as infants and another had died aged 6 in 1900. She devoted herself to her surviving children, Adolf and Paula. Klara was the third wife of Alois*

Hitler, a gruff and opinionated provincial civil servant, who had died in 1903. Adolf had despised his father and his father's way of life. Dr Bloch had never witnessed a 'closer attachment' between a mother and a son. Sadly, the doctor's examination revealed a fungating carcinoma of the breast.

The results of surgery alone on such locally advanced tumours are poor, because such tumours are inevitably already invading skin and the underlying muscle, meaning that surgical removal of all detectable tumour is impossible. However, we must remember that surgery alone was all that was available in 1907 to treat breast cancer. There was no chemotherapy or radiation therapy and there was little knowledge of breast cancer among the general population 100 years ago, most breast cancer patients at that time presented with either large breast masses or, as Klara Hitler did, when the mass started eating through the skin of the breast.

Appropriately, Dr. Bloch referred Klara Hitler to an unnamed Linz surgeon, who presumably performed an operation that was the standard of care at the time for breast cancer, a radical mastectomy. Unfortunately and not unexpectedly, Klara Hitler's tumour rapidly recurred on her chest wall by September 1907. Recurrences on the chest wall can be one of the most difficult clinical situations to deal with in breast cancer, particularly a local recurrence that keeps growing, fungating, and bleeding.

A number of scholars, such as the psychoanalyst Gertrude Kurth, proposed that Klara's suffering was the origin of Hitler's anti-Semitism. Kurth proposed that Hitler had "experienced a father-transference to the doctor" and ended up attributing "all positive traits to the doctor and … negative ones to the Jew," suggesting that Dr Bloch was responsible (in Hitler's mind) for the brutal assault and mutilation (by surgery) of his dear mother.

In 1941, Hitler personally ordered the removal of "the Jewish cancer" from the breast of Germany through the use of poison gas. Six million Jews died as a result. It is also of interest to note that one of the most potent icons of the Nazi era shows an heroic surgeon saving a damsel from the clutches of skeletal death i.e. the Aryan knight saving the Rhein Maiden from the Jewish cancer clutching her breast. (Figure 29)

****

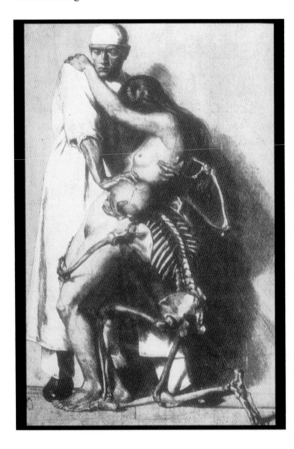

Fig. 29 The surgeon as Aryan knight saving the Rhine maiden from the clutches of death, Saliger 1936

In 1965 I passed the exams to become a Fellow of the Royal College of Surgeons (FRCS). As I floated up the grand staircase of the College in Lincoln's Inn Fields, to have my hand shaken by the then President, Lord Brock, I reflected on my luck in predicting a question on the rationale and technique of the radical *en bloc* technique for the cure of breast cancer.

I think it might be a fitting end to this chapter to describe the technique I mastered 40 years ago in full detail. [readers who feel faint at the description of surgery may feel free to skip this section]

To begin with I had to take a skin graft from the inner thigh of the patient so as not to be tempted to compromise on the surgical incision with closure of the wound in mind. This meant using an instrument like an old-fashioned cutthroat razor but about 30 cms in length. The slice of half thickness skin was taken with the same technique and skill as used by "fat Hymie" in our local delicatessen when cutting thin slices of fresh smoked salmon from a side of fish. This graft was then wrapped in moist saline gauze and placed on one side. Next I had to cut an ellipse of skin that included the nipple with at least 3.0 centimetres of skin in all directions from the palpable margins of the tumour. Don't ask me why 3.0 centimetres. The history of all radical surgery for all cancers is full of exhortations to take odd numbers of centimetres of normal tissue from the margins of the tumour. In retrospect this seems to have had more to do with the mystique of numerology than science! Next I had to undermine the skin flaps North and South so they were thin enough to transmit light like the finest porcelain, to avoid leaving a single cancer cell behind. Then starting at the clavicle I would cut down to the chest wall lifting a disc of tissue that incorporated the breast and the pectoralis major muscle separating it from its origin along the sternal edge. This flap containing the breast and underlying muscle was then reflected from the sternum across to the armpit, taking care to control the blood vessels that perforated the intercostal spaces feeding the breast from the internal mammary artery deep behind the sternum. Incorporated into this pound of flesh were the origins of the pectoralis minor that had to be cut by diathermy from its origin over the 2nd to the 5th ribs. All that was easy, although a little bit bloody. On average two pints of blood loss had to be anticipated by ordering blood from the bank the day before surgery. Then the tricky bit: identifying all the "clockwork" in the armpit (axilla). Starting at the first rib I learnt to identify the axillary vein, above which was the axillary artery and above that the cords of the brachial plexus that innervated the muscles of the arm and hand. One false move could lead to semi-paralysis. Following the lower margin along the axillary vein I had to identify and ligate all the tiny vessels that fed the breast as they disappeared into the fat of the axilla. One false move here might avulse a branch coming straight off the axillary vein that could add another pint to the tally for transfusion. Then all this fatty tissue that contained the all-important lymph nodes had to be brushed downwards off the muscle walls of the axilla to be incorporated *en bloc* with the whole "specimen". Next, deep in the axilla, lying on the subscapularis muscle I would identify the neurovascular bundle containing the nerve to latissimus dorsi. Damaging that would leave the patient with loss of power in the shoulder movements. Also deep in the axilla but lying on the chest wall I would need to find the "long nerve of Bell", a dainty nerve supplying the serratus anterior. Damaging that and the patient would

71

experience winging of the scapula every time she tried to push open a door. Finally the intercostal-brachial nerve would be seen adopting its curious bowstring course across the axilla to supply sensation to the under-surface of the arm. I was advised to sacrifice that nerve in the name of a radical cure, leaving the woman with quite disabling numbness and parasthaesia (pins and needles). Finally the skin on the lateral side of the operation was divided and the "specimen" dumped in a bucket for the pathologist to study in macroscopic and microscopic detail. After all the bleeding was stopped two drains were inserted and closure of the wound begins. If the wound was capable of being sutured together I had been insufficiently radical, so in most cases you closed what you could and covered the saucer shaped defect with the split skin graft taken at the start. The result was hideous not to mention the inevitable lymphoedema (swelling of the arm) that would follow as time progressed. The patient was then tightly bandaged and kept in hospital for an average of about ten days. God knows how she felt when the bandages were removed and she viewed this mutilation for the first time.

I've described this procedure in detail so that you can judge the starting point of my odyssey. Yet this procedure was "the treatment of choice" (oh how I hate that expression) for breast cancer all round the world until the mid 1970s. Even though I took some pride in my skills as a surgeon, I had a visceral disgust for the Halsted radical mastectomy. The story of its fall from favour will be recounted in the following chapters.

Chapter 6

The Natural History of Breast Cancer

Introduction

The expression "Natural History" has two meanings. Historically it has come to mean the systematic study of all natural objects, hence the famous collection of dinosaur skeletons, trilobite fossils and Darwin's specimens from the Galapagos Islands in the Natural History Museum, South Kensington, London.

Another meaning to this expression used as a medical term is the behaviour of a disease in the absence of treatment, or in other words *left to nature.*

In the modern world we accept the concept of the self-limiting nature of many mild ailments and jokingly reassure our friends that their bad cold will get better in a week, but with whiskey, a warm bed and tender loving care it will only take seven days.

With more serious conditions that are life-threatening or could lead to chronic dysfunction we treat in order to favourably influence this natural history and rely on the history books to tell us what would have happened in the absence of treatment but with careful observation alone. Unfortunately in the days before active treatment of serious disease, careful and systematic observation were also exceptional. And this applies in particular to carcinoma of the breast.

Another relevant issue here is that we don't ˇalways see in a dispassionate way the objective reality of that which we observe but more likely a distortion, refracted through the prism of our personal prejudices. Observations that reinforce our prejudices are embraced and those that challenge our beliefs are ignored or rationalized away.

But why should we have a prior set of beliefs, so powerful as to impair our observation of something so fundamental as the natural history of a life-threatening disease? The simple answer to that is "human nature".

Part of our success in evolution from the lower primates is the capacity to make order out of the myriad daily observations of our busy lives. We constantly but sub-consciously create hypotheses or models of objective reality – some are silly, many have a survival advantage and some in the fullness of time are found to have misled us.

Silly examples might include not stepping on the cracks between paving stones for fear of raising a demon. It works all the time! Such childlike beliefs persist in certain primitive societies who frighten away the dragon consuming the sun during an eclipse by banging drums and blowing horns – it never fails.

Conceptual models that have had a survival advantage might include the observation of wild animals and their feeding habits to decide what food is fit to eat or relating cloud formations to weather conditions to decide when to migrate or moor our boats. Misleading models of reality included the belief in the geocentric nature of the universe or the teachings of Karl Marx and Sigmund Freud.

However in this chapter I wish to concentrate on the natural history of breast cancer and the evolution of conceptual models to explain its behaviour. I propose that all this is fundamental to improving the lot of suffering patients for the simple reason that our treatments are the therapeutic consequence of our belief in the underlying mechanisms of disease. In other words belief systems and treatment modalities are two sides of the same coin.

The nature of models and models of nature

A model car we understand but a model of nature, what can that mean? Let me explain. Models are not just mechanical miniatures of the real thing; they can be anything else which helps to capture the very essence of the subject of our scrutiny. They can be metaphysical, mechanistic or mathematical, you can also throw in biological models of organic objects for good measure.

Let me illustrate this with two objects, one inorganic and the other organic.

Let us take that car we cherish so much. Many sports car enthusiasts keep perfect replicas scaled down to 1:1,000 on their desks in preference to photographs of their wives and children – for example my MGA referred to in chapter 4. This is a mechanical model. Their wives view the contraption as the work of the devil, i.e a metaphysical model. Finally the mechanical engineer can reproduce the energy of the internal combustion unit and the torque of the transmission system as mathematical formulae. That is a mathematical model.

My organic example is the rose bush I see from my study window and in particular one rose of an enchanting hue like the blush on the cheeks of Raphael's "Madonna with a Pomegranate."

"What's in a name? That which we call a rose by any other name would smell as sweet", is a Shakespearian metaphysical model of this organic object.

Dorothy Parker even provides me with a link between these two objects of desire:

"Why is it no one ever sent me yet
One perfect limousine, do you suppose?
Ah no, it's always just my luck to get
One perfect rose!"

Easier to handle is the mechanistic model in a child's primary school botany book. Here the rose is built up of petals, sepals, stamens, filament, anther and carpel all connected to a stalk with leaves, thorns and roots. It loses its poetry when broken down this way. Even more so you may think when the geneticists have their way and the rose is described as a molecular model. Curiously enough much of the beauty and mystery of the rose reappears in its mathematical model.

The new mathematics of Fibonacci numbers, fractals and Lindenmayer systems allow us to generate beautiful floribunda on our computer screens thus linking the mathematical model of the rose to the greater symmetries and complex patterns of all of God's creation.

The natural history of an automobile and of a rose

Left to nature an automobile will rust and its engine will seize up. As our knowledge of the automobile and of the mechanism of rusting developed in tandem we have a ready explanation for this process, which is well understood.

The chemical reaction between iron and oxygen in the presence of moisture leads to corrosion and the production of iron oxide (Fe_2O_3). (Furthermore our inner urban areas experience the miraculous transformation of our rubber tires into piles of bricks if left unattended for too long!.) We can influence this natural history by keeping the car dry, well oiled and locked away. With luck the automobile will now last us up to 20 years or more.

The rose has a different and much more complex natural history. Left to nature it will enjoy an annual cycle of renewal, flowering every summer, resting every winter and springing into bud each spring. In addition it grows into angry knots, it develops suckers with seven leaves instead of five on each stem, which grow to prodigious lengths. Then holes appear in the leaves, brown patches of rust add to their disfigurement and green or black creepy crawlies infest and destroy the buds. In the bad old days you could accuse your neighbour of witchcraft for blighting your bushes (a metaphysical model of disease) but in this modern era we know that the "rust" is a fungus (*Puccinia basdiomycetes*) and the holes are thanks to the caterpillars. I can influence this natural history with the aid of scientific horticulture, by pruning in February, putting phosphates down in March and spraying with ***non-organic chemicals*** all summer. ("Organic roses" are a mess!) This way the expectation of life of a rose bush can be 40 years with blooms as big as cabbages, adding lustre to our lives.

Breast Cancer

After that long preamble, the relevance of which will soon become clear, I wish to return to the natural history of breast cancer. If left untreated what would happen and why?

To start with I wish to describe two anecdotal case histories, one from the 17th century and one from the 21st.

As mentioned in the previous chapter, the Louvre, Paris houses a large and beguiling masterpiece by Rembrandt, "Bathsheba at her toilet". Completed in 1655, the painting shows a naked Bathsheba looking wistfully into the middle distance left, whilst holding a letter in her right hand. Her attendant bathes her feet in a pool and the background is dark and ambiguous. Perhaps she has just learnt of her husband's death in battle as a result of King David's treachery, leaving her free to join the long list of the royal concubines. About 25 years ago whilst working as a senior lecturer in the department of surgery at the Welsh National School of Medicine in Cardiff, a young Australian research fellow, Peter Braithwaite, drew my attention to the dimple in the upper outer quadrant of Bathsheba's left breast. I had to agree with him, the model for this painting has the classical stigma of breast cancer, which I have confirmed on subsequent visits to the Louvre to see the painting in the flesh, so to speak. I encouraged him to research the history of the painting and its model. His work on this ultimately appeared in print, since when Bathsheba has become an icon of the breast cancer movement. In short the model was Hendrekje Stoffels who doubled up as mistress and housekeeper for Rembrandt. She was in her thirties when the picture was completed and died eight years later. Her mode of dying was characteristic of breast cancer with secondaries to the liver. There is no record of her being treated, but in any case treatment in those days was a futile hocus pocus based on the doctrines of Aristotle and Galen, yet she lived a further eight years after the clinically obvious disease, unknowingly portrayed in the painting, became apparent.

More recently a woman booked into my clinic at the Portland hospital, as an "old patient", yet my secretary had no record of her. It transpired that I had seen her on only one occasion and that was eight years previously at The Royal Marsden Hospital. Piecing the story together I suddenly recalled the visit. She was 49 at the time but was now 57. I had diagnosed multi-focal carcinoma of the left breast at biopsy and recommended a mastectomy to be followed by 5 years of tamoxifen. She firmly but politely declined my advice and as she put it, placed herself in the hands of Jesus and the prayers of her evangelical community. Not believing in the power of prayer to heal (almost no one dies of breast cancer without an attempt at intercessionary prayer) I confessed to surprise at seeing her alive and wanted to know how I could help. The only complaint to which she confessed was swelling of the left arm. Exchanging glances with her attentive husband and daughter I asked her to disrobe in the examination room, bracing myself for the worst. Well it wasn't the worst I've seen but it was pretty gruesome nonetheless. Both breasts were now replaced by hard nodules of cancer and both axillae (armpits) were full of the disease causing massive lymphoedema (swelling due to the accumulation of tissue fluid) of the arms, yet there was no evidence of distant metastases. Not wishing to push my luck too far by asking for another biopsy I made the assumption that the tumour was hormone responsive and advised to start on anastrozole (Arimidex – see chapter 12) suggesting that Jesus now needed a little help from modern medicine as prayer alone would no longer hold the cancer in check.

She politely took my prescription and promised to return in one month to check on progress. Needless to say she failed to keep that appointment. In Rembrandt's day that might not have been such a bad idea, but in the modern world, I would judge it irresponsible behaviour. One must not laugh at such profound faith but I know that much of the suffering she can expect before she dies could have been avoided.

Two anecdotes don't make a summary so just how typical are these examples?

Breast cancer in the 19th and early 20th century

In 1970 whilst working with Dr Bernard Fisher in Pittsburgh, I visited the library of the National Institute of Health (NIH) in Bethesda with the object of completing an historical review for my thesis. Whilst searching for one reference a more important one literally fell in my lap, (a process us scholars describe as library gremlins at play). This happened to be a treatise on breast cancer by one Dr. Gross of Philadelphia published in 1880. Latterly I've recognized that this was the same Dr. Gross immortalized in Thomas Eakins' masterpiece, "The Gross clinic", which I was fortunate to see in an exhibition at the Metropolitan Museum of Art in New York the summer of 2004. (Figure 30)

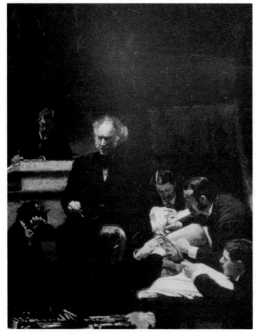

Fig. 30 The Gross clinic by Thomas Eakins

This is a large dark and brooding painting which shows the great surgeon at work treating a young man for osteomyelitis (a chronic infection) of the femur. The surgeon is highlighted wearing his frock coat with the sleeves turned back, assistants hold the boy down, the anaesthetic is rag and bottle chloroform, the boy's mother looks on in anguish whilst within a dimly lit amphitheatre a group of students look on with rapt attention.

I had always admired this painting in reproduction and was surprised that Dr Gross had a passing interest in breast cancer. Paradoxically Eakins' other great surgical tableau, the "Guthrie clinic", also seen in New York, shows a mastectomy operation near completion with another great surgeon, Dr Guthrie, standing back in dramatic pose flourishing his scalpel like an artist's brush whilst his humble assistant closes the skin. (Figure 31) Ah! Those were the days: I was born 100 years too late. But I digress.

Gross' treatise provides a clear insight into the status of the disease in the era immediately before the period when the developments in anaesthesia and antisepsis allowed surgeons to attempt a radical cure of breast cancer. He describes a series of 616 cases, most of which had skin infiltration on presentation which had ulcerated through in 25% of the patients. About two thirds had extensive involvement of axillary nodes (glands in the armpit). Accepting that the meagre benefits of surgery seldom outweighed the risks in those days, he

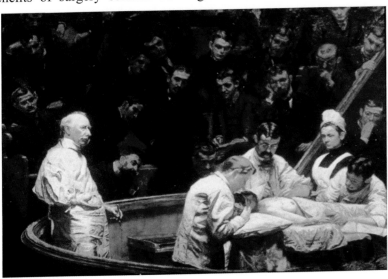

Fig. 31 The Guthrie clinic by Thomas Eakins

judged it ethical to follow the natural course of 97 cases that received nothing other than "constitutional support".

He describes how skin ulcers appeared on average 20 months after a tumour is first detected, with growth into the chest wall itself after a further two months, and direct invasion of the other breast if the patient lived on average three years after the lump first appeared. A quarter of all these untreated cases went on to develop obvious secondaries in vital organs within a year and another quarter after three years. In the end only one in twenty survived more than 5 years.

Since then a number of different series of untreated breast cancer have been reported. For example one report in 1926 described over 600 cases of untreated breast cancer with only 60 remaining alive at the end of 10 years. Another in 1927 described a series of 100 patients who were considered inoperable, unfit for surgery or who had refused the offer of surgery. The average duration of life was 4 years for the whole group.

The study that has attracted the most attention over the years was that of the great oncologist Dr. Julian Bloom published in 1968. His data came from the records of 250 women dying of breast cancer in the Middlesex Hospital Cancer ward between 1905 and 1933. It should be noted that almost all of them presented with neglected disease, many already with secondaries in vital organs. The survival rates from the "alleged onset" of symptoms were 5% at 5 years with only two alive at 15 years. The reasons for withholding treatment are also worthy of note: most of them were too old or infirm to withstand treatment and 20% refused treatment.

Although of historical interest I can't really believe that these studies help to provide a baseline against which to judge the curative effect of modern treatment. Firstly, as with all retrospective reports there has to be an element of selection; why was treatment withheld? It is quite obvious that in the majority of these cases, with the exception of those refusing treatment, they all had an exceptionally poor prognosis to begin with. Secondly, they mostly represent women seeking medical attention at a time in the late 19thC or early 20thC, when many women were content to co-exist with their lump in blissful ignorance until they died of old age or were knocked down by a horse and carriage. Next, the accuracy of the diagnosis might be called into question in the days before modern microscopy.

Finally, for all we know the biological nature of the disease might have changed over the last 50 years as the incidence has increased following the major upheavals after the second world war, life style changes that include delaying the first pregnancy, obesity due to cheaper and more plentiful food and the widespread adoption of the oral contraceptive pill and HRT.

It would of course be inconceivable to suggest we study an untreated group today and the closest approximation we can find comes from a report of the Ontario cancer clinics between 1938 and 1956, just preceding the jump in breast cancer incidence in the developed world. Close on 10,000 cases were analyzed in the province of Ontario during this period. Amongst this group were 150 well-documented cases who received no treatment of any kind. Although, yet again 100 of these cases were untreated because of late stage of presentation or poor general condition, the rest were unable or unwilling to attend for treatment. A careful note was made of the date the patient first became aware of the lump from which point survival rates were computed. About a third survived for 5 years from first recorded symptom and the average survival of the whole group was 4 years. The most surprising figure was a near 70% 5 year survival for the small group presenting with truly early disease! Let me emphasise that – nearly three-quarters of those diagnosed with the type of breast cancer we see today in the Western world *survived 5 years without treatment*. However we can't quantify the *quality of* that *survival*.

The influence of surgery on the natural history of breast cancer

From the popularization of the classical radical mastectomy at the very end of the 19thC until about 1975 almost all patients with breast cancer of a technically operable stage were treated with modifications of the radical mastectomy. To those without commitment to a prior hypothesis, this allowed for new insights into the nature of the malignant process. Before considering this matter it's worth revisiting the conceptual model that allowed the radical operation to reign supreme for 75 years.

In about 1840, Dr. Rudolph Virchow of Berlin, the founding father of the discipline of pathology, described a revolutionary model of the disease building on the development of microscopy and postmortem examinations of the cadavers of breast cancer victims. He suggested that the disease started as a single focus within the breast, expanding with time and then migrating along lymphatic channels to the lymph glands in the axilla. These glands were said to act as a first line of defence filtering out the cancer cells. Once these filters became saturated the glands themselves acted as a nidus for tertiary spread to a second and then third line of defence like the curtain walls around a medieval citadel. Ultimately when all defences were exhausted the disease spread along tissue planes to the skeleton and vital organs.

The therapeutic consequences of this belief had to await the development of anaesthesia and antisepsis in the 1880s but were seized upon by Halsted in about 1895. William S. Halsted of the Johns Hopkins Hospital, Baltimore, was a very interesting man and a great surgical pioneer. He was a dapper gentleman who sent his shirts to London for laundering! In later life he became an opium addict but is best remembered for his pioneering work in postgraduate surgical education. Incidentally he invented the surgeon's rubber glove although this was not in the name of antisepsis but in the name of love. He fell in love with his beautiful scrub nurse who then developed allergic dermatitis on her hands in response to the carbolic acid used for antisepsis at the time. The rubber gloves were to protect her hands whilst she continued to assist him.

Armed with the teachings of Virchow, the developments in anaesthesia and antisepsis and prodigious surgical skills, it seemed inevitable that his patients would be cured by radical operations that cut away all of the breast, the overlying skin, the underlying muscles and as many lymph node groups compatible with the patients' survival.

So convincing were his arguments and so charismatic their chief proponent, the Halsted operation was adopted as default therapy all round the world.

At this long perspective we are entitled to ask to what extent did the radical operation add to the curability of the disease and what can we learn about the nature of the beast by its behaviour following such mutilating surgery?

We can also add a third question concerning human nature and our unwillingness to see facts "which almost slap us in the face".*

William Halsted operated at a time when the triumph of mechanistic principles was at its peak when the common man had begun enjoying the fruits of the Industrial Revolution. Naturally, Halsted's 'complete operation' was based on mechanistic concepts about the nature of cancer.

(*"*It is now, as it was then, as it may ever be, conceptions from the past blind us to facts which almost slap us in the face*" – WS Halsted 1908)

His surgical expertise was remarkable, and for the first time, breast cancer seemed curable with recurrence rates of only 10% at 3 years, very low compared to the other series at that time. Halsted's pioneering work in breast cancer served as a model for many other solid cancers and his principles are still successful for cancers of the head and neck, the "commando operation", and cervix, the "Wertheim operation".

Unfortunately, only about a quarter of patients treated by Halsted survived 10 years. The natural reaction to this failure was not to question the belief in the centrifugal spread of cancer, but to attempt even more radical treatment. Internal mammary lymph nodes under the sternum (breast bone) that receive about 25% of the lymphatic drainage from the breast were not removed in Halsted's 'complete operation' but were included in the super radical operations that were fashionable in the 1940–1960 era. Alternatively attempts to kill off these hypothetical residual foci of the disease were made by including them in the fields of radiation after surgery.

All this achieved was to increase peri-operative deaths and add a swollen arm (lymphoedema) to the gross disfigurement of the chest wall with no improvement in cure rate. Thus even when the tumour seemed to have been completely 'removed with its roots', the patients still developed distant metastases and succumbed: about half of all patients eventually dying of the disease over 10 years and with no evidence of "cure" if patients were followed up for 25 years. For example a seminal study by Diana Brinkley and John Haybittle, published in the Lancet in 1975, described a group of over 700 breast cancer patients treated by radical surgery in Addenbrooke's Hospital Cambridge and followed up for 25 years. They continued to demonstrate an excess mortality compared to a population matched for age and this excess mortality was principally related to breast cancer that continued to recur (in spite of it " all being taken away") for the complete period of follow up. This could mean only one thing – "shutting the stable door after the horse had bolted".

The biological revolution of the late 20th century

Prompted by the failures of radical operations to cure patients with breast cancer, Professor Bernard Fisher from Pittsburgh PA (my mentor) proposed a revolutionary hypothesis that rejected the mechanistic model of the past, replacing it with a biological model based on ten years' painstaking work with laboratory mice which challenged and refuted every prediction from the time of Virchow. From these animal experiments he postulated that cancer spreads via the blood stream first of all, bypassing the lymphatic channels, and that this can occur even before the lump is first detectable: The rate of growth and the rate of spread being determined by the nature of the beast at its inception. Aggressive (poorly differentiated) cancers, growing and spreading rapidly and indolent (well differentiated) cancers, doing the same at a pace measured in years rather than months. Furthermore, Fisher speculated that the patient is not a passive host to the disease, but has the capacity to mount a defence against its incursion via cell-mediated immunity triggered within the lymph glands themselves. Putting this all together he argued that the outcome of treatment by surgery alone was pre-determined by the biology of tumour–host interactions. Indirect evidence of success or failure of this battle could be deduced by the status of the glands at surgery. Negative (uninvolved) nodes might suggest an intact host defence whilst positive (involved) nodes represented an exhausted system that has allowed the cancer cells to maraud unchecked around the body. Or to put it succinctly: involved glands in the axilla are the expression rather than determinant of a poor prognosis.

I've coined the term 'biological predeterminism' to describe this theory, from which one can make the following predictions:

(A)   The extent of local treatment by surgery and radiotherapy might control the disease on the chest wall but have no effect on survival, the horse (cancer) having bolted before the stable door (radical surgery) was slammed shut.

(B)   If the outcome of treatment was pre-determined by the extent of microscopic (occult) secondaries present at the time of diagnosis, then the only chance of cure would be with so called adjuvant systemic therapy i.e. drugs targeting these putative sites of disease, for patients with even localized tumours. These drugs could then be selected from those known to produce responses in advanced disease such as a combination of cytotoxic agents (chemotherapy) or drugs which could interfere with production or uptake of oestrogens by the tumour (hormone therapy). (see chapter 12)

As regards the extent of local treatment, many trials have tested less versus more surgery with or without post-operative radiotherapy.

A recent world overview of these trials concluded that more radical local treatment does not have any influence on the appearance of distant disease or overall survival with one caveat. This is in spite of the increase in local recurrence rates with less radical local treatment, i.e. although radical surgery or postoperative radiotherapy has a substantial effect on reducing local recurrence rates, it doe not improve overall survival. Furthermore, as predicted, breast cancer survival can be influenced favourably with adjuvant systemic therapy.

All the above can be taken as powerful corroboration of Fisher's theory that metastases of any importance have already occurred *before* the clinical or radiological detection of most breast cancers.

Fisher's theories so influenced my philosophy concerning the future direction of breast cancer research that in 1970 I took myself off to Pittsburgh to work in his laboratory and from there embarked on a career in clinical research for the treatment of this terrible disease.

In the next chapter I want to describe my experiences during this seminal time in the USA and then go on to describe how the teachings of the great philosopher, Sir Karl Popper (who was to become my friend during the last few years of his life) translated the "logic of scientific discovery" into hard facts that contributed to a near 50% reduction in breast cancer mortality within the last 20 years.

Chapter 7

Pittsburgh 1970–1971

Every ambitious British academic believes that to advance in your career you need the qualification BTA. This stands for "been to America". I was no different but in my defence, as I've already explained, I was of the opinion that only one guy in the world was making any sense in the study of breast cancer and that was Dr. Bernard Fisher of the Presbyterian Hospital, Pittsburgh, PA. I was therefore very keen to take a sabbatical and work with the man who was making the waves. Judy was very supportive, providing those waves were off the Pacific, Orange County, CA, or second choice fairly close to 5ᵗʰ Avenue, New York, NY. But Pittsburgh! Everybody said it was the pits and to escape from Newcastle upon slag heaps to Pittsburgh upon slag heaps was too cruel. However I prevailed on the condition that we visited Saks 5ᵗʰ Avenue, New York, NY whilst overseas.

So I packed my bag and Judy packed her 7 bags and Richard packed his bag and Katie packed her 4 bags and then there were the brown paper carrier bags for the teddy bears and dolls that had to be carry-on luggage as well as the drinks and games and other paraphernalia that were apparently obligatory when travelling with two children aged 6 and 4. The brown paper bags split en route and little Katie walked up and down the Boeing, up and down and up and down. In fact we could have walked to the States by the time we arrived. We were very pleasantly surprised on arrival in Pittsburgh. Apparently with the closure of much of the coal industry and many of the steel mills, the city had enjoyed a renaissance, and (apart from the polluted air) was really quite beautiful in the vivid colours of the maples in their full autumnal glory.

Pittsburgh sits in a triangle of land boarded by the three rivers at the point where the Ohio splits into the Alleghany and Monongahela. At the apex of this junction there was the giant three-river stadium that housed the Steelers (American football) in the winter and the Pirates (baseball, a girly kind of game like rounders) in the summer. As you moved further north east from downtown the land became more and more hilly and sported many beautiful gardens and parks. Most of the heavy industry was close to the waters of the Monongahela with the suburbs tasting the pollution only if the wind blew from the southwest. As you exited the tunnel through Mount Washington on the way in from the airport and looked down on the city and its three rivers the view was breathtaking – either the burnt umber of the fall, the white of the winter or the rich greens of the spring/summer.

Dr. Fisher's lovely wife Shirley, (still beautiful if somewhat disabled in her 80s when visited last year), took us under her wing and set about finding us living accommodation. This was the first of many extraordinary demonstrations of friendliness and generosity we experienced in the USA.

First off we went to visit the ranch-style palace of the senior vice president of Westinghouse. Shirley played tennis with the wife and they were looking for "house sitters" for a year whilst the husband was seconded abroad. This was on offer free providing we looked after the place. The double doors opened onto an atrium with thick-pile pale pink carpets that came up to the medial malleolus of my ankle.

There was one set of stairs going up and another set of stairs going down. Judy was rather taken by the walk-in fridge and the third tap in the kitchen that provided water already boiling. I was rather taken by the basement that resembled a London gentleman's club with a games room and a fully stocked bar. The kids were rather taken with the rare porcelain all within easy reach of their sticky fingers. I was then reminded of Baum's third law of thermodynamics that goes something like this.... In any meta-stable system the rate of entropy accelerates directly to the power of the number of children of the age of 5 or under, squared. A house with thick-pile pink carpets and porcelain within easy reach counts as such a system. We therefore with great regret declined the kind offer, and eventually settled in a modest two-bedroom apartment on Walnut Street, Shadyside.

We visited there last year when I was a guest speaker at a conference to find that Shadyside was the "in" place, a bit like Upper Street, Islington, although back in 1970 it was quiet and sedate.

Once settled Richard entered kindergarten and Katie shopped with Judy doing "cute" for England. The Americans were totally disarmed by this pretty little four year old speaking with a cut-glass English accent and lavished cookies and candy on her. She caught on quickly and started to exaggerate her accent until we translated cookies and candy into English, meaning premature tooth rot. (Figure 32)

I then went off to meet the boss.

Bernie was a large craggily handsome American stereotype, or so I thought. (Figure 33) As it turned out he was also Jewish. (Remember what I wrote about my father-in-law and the chameleon characteristic of my race?) What I hadn't expected was to be mentored by two Fisher

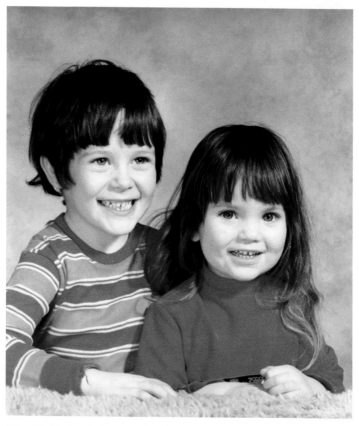

Fig. 32 Richard & Katie Pittsburgh 1971

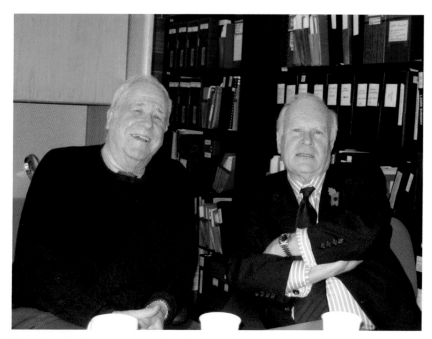

Fig. 33 Dr. Fisher and me Pittsburgh 2006

brothers. The younger, Ed Fisher, was a world-renowned pathologist living on a very short fuse scaring the living daylights out of me. He sacked his long suffering PA every week but seemed to tolerate me, providing the best tuition in pathology I've experienced and to this day I can hold my own in any clinico-pathology conference with the best of them. I made one faux pas though that nearly destroyed our relationship.

Unbeknownst to me, the younger Edwin Fisher had been a promising college baseball player who once considered playing for the Pittsburgh Pirates rather than a career in pathology.

He was not amused by my tired old joke about it being a girly game. Having been taken by him to watch the Pirates at play I realized that it was a brutal game, played by men wearing long johns facing a stone hard ball being propelled at 120 mph at their face without a bounce. I found it very boring although I loved the marching bands and pom-pom girls.

There is a kind of machismo amongst American surgeons, not only do they swagger like the old gunslingers of the wild west, but they try to outdo each other with the early start to the day. As a result I would join the cleaning staff on the tramcar each morning at 5.00am in order to be there in good time to collect the blood specimens before the chief did his rounds at 6.00am in order to start in the OR at 7.00am. Those of us who gained a BTA tried to introduce these habits into the NHS on return with little success. I used to sit gowned and gloved in the operating theatre at King's College Hospital for a start time of 8.30 am watching with increasing frustration as the rest of the staff would drift in yawning, with "knife to skin" delayed for three-quarters of an hour. Come 12.00 mid-day theatre sister would insist that I cancelled the last case so that her staff could have lunch before the afternoon list.

I loved the camaraderie in the OR and even on the first day the chief of orthopaedic surgery, who was an Anglophile, said that we must come round to dinner. Now in truth in England when a stranger you meet says, "you must come round for dinner", that's the last you ever hear from them. Yet on the first evening after this encounter Judy was waiting to tell me that we all had an invite for dinner next Saturday, including the kids, at the absurdly early hour of 5.00pm. It appeared that to compensate for these early starts they ate early in the evening. That next weekend we dressed the kids in cute and overdressed ourselves in British, to arrive "fashionably late" at 5.30pm; an alien concept in the USA.

To enter the palatial mansion we had to circumnavigate a very strange shaped swimming pool. On enquiry we learnt that the pool was the shape of the femoral bone and the diving board at the circular end of the long shaft was in the exact anatomical place of the *ligamentum teres*. The Americans feel no shame in exhibiting their wealth and are also anxious to illustrate from whence their wealth was derived.

We were served a delicious fruit punch and Judy asked for seconds. I wandered round the incredibly warm and friendly gathering summoned on our behalf, whilst the womenfolk oohed and aahed as the kids performed their English "cute" act.

I enquired as to the nature of this delicious fruit punch only to learn that they were whiskey sours based on Tennessee bourbon whiskey. By the time I caught up with the wife it was too late, she was now having a wow of a time and totally disinhibited.

This is now our staple drink on our many visits to the USA and it always reminds us of yet another striking example of American hospitality.

Enough digression. Let me get back to the main reason for this visit to Pittsburgh.

I embarked on two scientific projects that explored the Fisherian hypothesis concerning the nature of breast cancer. The first was in the laboratory and the second in the clinical trials office. This alone illustrated the genius of Bernie Fisher in that in parallel he was running laboratory experiments to understand the biological nature of the disease whilst running large scale clinical trials to test these insights gained from experimental mice into clinical practice for women with breast cancer.

I will return to this theme when describing my philosophy of science in a later chapter.

My lab work continued on the lines I had set up at King's in the hope that it would lead to a thesis and higher degree. In those days it was fashionable to believe that the body mounted a natural immune response to cancer that protected the body in health but once exhausted allowed cancers to progress unchecked. This concept is still fashionable amongst the proponents of alternative medicine to this day. A major component of the immune response to foreign cellular material (cell mediated immunity as distinct to humoural immunity that is activated in response to vaccines) is the monocyte/macrophage system. Macrophage literally means "big eaters", that is why I've always felt a sense of shared affinity with them. These ubiquitous cells, also known as phagocytes, were much favoured by the fictional character of Sir Ralph Bloomfield-Bonnington in Shaw's "The Doctor's Dilemma". "There is only one sure way to cure all disease and that is to stimulate the phagocytes". These cells were known to be first in line to ingest and process cellular debris, in order to present the foreign antigens to the lymphocyte population that then kickstarted a cascade of events that sent scavenger cells circulating round the body to seek and destroy these foreign invaders. I mastered a very delicate technique of harvesting bone marrow from mice and culturing the material in such a way that the precursor cells of the monocyte/macrophage system grew in colonies in the soft agar culture dishes. The number of these colonies reflected the state of activation of this cellular lineage at the time of harvest. I then set up controlled experiments with colonies of syngeneic mice, all of them effectively being identical twins. Some were left untreated, others had injections of a suspension of mouse mammary cancers that had developed in the same colony, and the third had sham injections. The fact that the mice were all inbred meant that any biological response could not be due to the body recognizing "non-self" cellular material but had to be due to transformations on the cancer cell surface that tricked the mouse's immune system into thinking there were alien invaders around. The results were spectacular in that the colony count for the mice with breast cancers growing on their flanks shot up whilst nothing happened in the control groups. This was reasonably interpreted that the body could react at a distance to cellular debris shed from the surface of a growing cancer and that, switched on, the first step of a cell mediated immune response. The clinical corollary to this might be the use of non-specific vaccines that might stimulate the phagocytes and act as an adjuvant therapy to enhance the outcome of surgery alone. Sad to say that this approach (that became very popular in France in the early 1970s) failed to deliver and I had to wait for nearly 30 years before the significance of my findings became apparent. Unfortunately by then my experimental findings had been long forgotten and rightly so.

My work in the clinical trials office however was to bear fruit of lasting value.

At that time Bernie's clinical trials collaborative, the National Surgical Adjuvant Breast Project (NSABP) was in its relative infancy. They were currently running their fourth protocol that was rather unimaginatively referred to as B04. Not surprisingly the design of the study was based on the same biological principles as the King's/Cambridge trial I described in the last chapter. However in this case the comparisons were between cases of breast cancer treated in a surgically conventional way, mastectomy plus a radical clearance of the axillary lymph nodes (ALN) compared with mastectomy alone, with the lymph nodes left intact and treatment delayed if their progression became a problem. Although simple in design the question posed challenged the central tenet of the radical school of thought. If failure to treat the ALN resulted in a worse prognosis then Halsted was right and the invaded ALN did indeed form a nidus for tertiary spread of the disease. If the outcome was the other way round then Fisher was right and the intact ALN were important in mounting an immune response to the cancer. Just like the King's/Cambridge trial, the long term results showed no difference in survival whatsoever but at least supported Fisher's assertion that the involved ALN were the expression of the poor prognosis rather than its determinant. From our modern standpoint we take this as a given, however at the time it was considered either revolutionary or heretical. The King's/Cambridge trial added another fascinating insight about which I will tease the reader until full disclosure in chapter 9.

Sadly before my time was up Professor Murray summoned me back to London and it was with great regret that we repacked our bags that had, by a process known as parthenogenesis, increased in number since our arrival, and returned home. Unrecognized at the time, Judy was also carrying additional baggage that resulted in us welcoming a little Welsh girl into our family within the next six months.

Chapter 8

Cardiff 1972–1979

Shortly after returning to England I was appointed senior lecturer in the department of surgery at the University Hospital of Wales in Cardiff. In British academic medical hierarchy, a senior lecturer has the rank of an honorary consultant surgeon to the NHS and the equivalent of assistant professor at the university. I was only 35, which was young by the standards of the time. We were very excited by this move, all the more so when we noted the differential of house prices between London and Cardiff.

For what we got in the sale of our tiny tacky town house in Forest Hill, south east London, we could afford a mansion in Cardiff. As we were expecting our third child by then, the chance of another bedroom was most welcome. Judy fell in love at first sight with a grand detached house in Cyn Coed Road in the smartest suburb in town. I was in a state of shock when I was shown the magnificent rose gardens and terraced lawns back and front and estimated the time it would take to maintain the gardens whilst working in my *spare time* as a surgeon. This time Judy prevailed on the understanding that on my weekends off duty I would tend the gardens. There is an old saying in South Wales that if you can see the mountains it's going to rain and if you can't see the mountains it's already raining. It always seemed to rain on my weekends off duty!

It was a lovely house though, the best we ever owned, and I paid dearly for this privilege on our return to London seven years later.

Those seven years in Cardiff were amongst the happiest of our lives. We rapidly made friends with the locals who were warm and hospitable. We loved the Welsh for their mellifluous accent, their singing voices, their mountains and their rugby. Shortly after settling in our beautiful, blonde and bouncing baby Welsh girl, Suzanne, was born to us.

It's a sobering thought that as I write this, 37 years later, my little Welsh girl has just delivered her third baby and our ninth grandchild.

The University Hospital of Wales (UHW) was a magnificent new building that also housed the medical school. It was the first and last time in my career that I was working in a half decent NHS facility, as most of the others had seen better days as Victorian work-houses. Mind you we still had to deal with all the emergencies that were admitted to The Royal Victoria Infirmary (RVI) in the centre of town. True to form all its walls were covered in the cream and brown tiles that have haunted my surgical career in the NHS.

My new boss was Professor Les Hughes, an Australian, one of the most gifted surgeons I had ever known. Unlike the *laisser faire* of my previous boss, Professor Hughes ran a tight ship. We had a huge department with magnificent operating theatres and laboratories. The theatres had viewing galleries for visitors and one of our anaesthetists who was a bit of a wag would hold up a placard with the word APPLAUSE printed in large capitals for the students in the gallery whenever I did something that looked impressive. In those days I was what used to be known as a general surgeon. Like most of my colleagues I lived by the infamous aphorism governing the three indications for surgery. Number one: We had seen someone do the procedure and fancied having a go ourselves. Number two: We'd done it before and rather enjoyed doing it. Number three: The patient actually needed the operation. Although half in jest there is no doubt that I really enjoyed the satisfaction of a major procedure well done and would often get to bed in the early hours with my underwear saturated in blood (to the disgust of my long suffering wife), yet with a sense of blissful self-fulfilment. Although many surgical procedures look difficult and daunting, once you've mastered the basic manoeuvres of the craft they are relatively easy to perform. For example a radical oesophago-gastrectomy for cancer at the junction of the gullet and the stomach, whilst looking dramatic, with an oblique incision opening the chest and the upper abdomen from the tip of the left clavicle to the umbilicus, was in fact an easy technical feat if you had a good eye, steady hands and a bit of *chutzpah*. In contrast much more challenging and scary were those cases where you had to preserve tiny nerve filaments whose division would be catastrophic and might end with you in the law courts. Two examples come to mind, thyroidectomy and superficial parotidectomy. Large goitres were common in the Welsh valleys, and finding the filamentous recurrent laryngeal nerve supplying the larynx (voice box) deep in the groove between the trachea and gullet, whilst holding onto a thyroid gland the size of a grapefruit, was a bit of an ordeal. One slip and the best tenor in the Caerphilly miners male voice choir would croak for the rest of his life. Even worse was a parotidectomy. The parotid is the major salivary gland that sits upon the angle of the jaw. Benign tumours in this gland can grow to prodigious proportions and if neglected turn malignant. Bad luck for us surgeons was the fact that the five branches of the facial nerve run right through the centre of the gland. These neural twigs have the calibre of the gossamer thread spiders employ to create their intricate webs. One false move and the corner of the mouth will never smile again, two false moves and an eyelid will droop for ever, three false moves…well you've got the picture by now. In retrospect one of the attractions of breast surgery as a speciality is the fact that the nerves you have to preserve are quite easy to find and avoid.

We enjoyed a lively common room in the department of surgery and in most break intervals you would find a group of us enjoying a lively debate about the nature and treatment of cancer. One of the enduring friendships I made then was with the young John Forbes, an Australian surgeon on a sabbatical. He and I shared the same sense of fun and also shared the reputation of being iconoclasts. He followed a parallel career path to mine and ended up professor of surgery in Newcastle NSW and director of the ANZ collaborative clinical trials group that pooled data with my own group from the 1980s onwards. Later on in our careers and in the company of our wives, we would share many adventures fulfilling our duty as world class "onco-tourists".

The majority of us young guns were persuaded of the veracity of the Fisherian heresy, but not our head of department. Les Hughes continued to practise the classical radical mastectomy until his retirement. In a way this is interesting. Les was a kindly man, a well-read scholar and a good surgeon, but he just didn't "get it". This observation more or less confirms that what we were witnessing was a true conceptual revolution or "paradigm shift" and if you won't look out of the box you will never see what lies beyond its walls. (see also chapter 19)

One of my younger colleagues for a time was something of a celebrity. JPR Williams, the greatest rugby union full back of all time, who played for Wales in the heady years of the 1970s, acted as my registrar for 6 months. His fame and his height rather eclipsed me as his nominal chief but at least through this connection I was never short of a ticket for the big games at Cardiff Arms Park. I watched Wales win the grand slam or the Triple Crown again and again. I even watched the greatest game of all time when the Barbarians beat the All-Blacks in 1977. My own claim to fame at Cardiff Arms Park came in the first ten minutes of the Welsh Rugby Union cup final in 1973 when Cardiff were playing Llanelli, when a voice suddenly boomed from the tannoy, "would Mr Baum go immediately to the RVI". I jumped out of my seat and got to the nearby hospital in no time at all. I remember the case clearly as an elderly man haemorrhaging from an ulcerated gastric cancer. I was able to resect the stomach and save his life only for him to die with recurrent disease less than a year later. In fact an early observation of mine on starting work in South Wales was just how common stomach cancer was compared with London. I even published a paper on this with the department of epidemiology that confirmed that the incidence of gastric cancer was indeed abnormally high in the mining valleys. I went as far as to suggest that the miners, ingesting carbon and silica with their sandwiches, might have contributed to their disease. Interestingly enough gastric cancer has almost disappeared now since the mines have closed, so the theory might not have been too far fetched.

I loved teaching the Welsh boys and girls and this love was reciprocated when I was elected as honorary president of the student's union. My role was to preside over the annual St. David's Day dinner and ball and to entertain the student's executive in my home. On those occasions after a drink or three, the students would organize themselves into spontaneous choirs, singing in rich harmony, "bread of heaven" and "*sospan fach*". They tended to drink me out of house and home and once in desperation they discovered where I kept the *Kiddush* (sacramental) wine and polished that off as well. Anyone who has ever tasted Palwin no. 10 will understand how desperate they must have been.

One of my more successful innovations for teaching the undergraduates started off as a joke. Traditionally teaching clinical skills to medical undergraduates has been on the basis of "the firm". The firm consisted of two or three consultants, a senior registrar, a junior registrar and the house officer. All were involved in the teaching of a group of between 6 to 10 students. The students were attached to us in three monthly blocks and we all bonded. At the end of the block the students would organize a "firm party" and compete with each other in their hospitality (if only to make up for poor grades) with fine cuisine and fine wines. At the end of one firm the students presented me with a rather cheeky gift. It was a plaster caste of a hand gilded with sparkly paint. The hand had the index finger extended and slightly bent whilst the other three fingers were tightly curled into the palm. This is the position the hand adopts when you are taught to do a rectal examination the correct way. I then had the bright idea of mounting the hand on a wooden plaque that carried an engraved plate bearing the title, "Golden Finger Award".

This award was to be won in a case presentation competition between the surgical firms.

A case presentation was a form of assessment whereby a pair of students would adopt a patient and follow them through their therapeutic journey. At the end of the firm they would present the case to the assembled group describing presentation, clinical and radiological examinations, diagnosis, treatment and pathology, finishing off with a discussion on the disease and the current literature. Often these were polished performances and an excellent teaching aid for the other students. The idea of "The Golden Finger Award" was to mobilize the latent rivalry between the surgical firms so that they competed against each other in addition to earning brownie points for their assessments. Right from the start it was a great success and when the Dean got to learn about it he insisted that the whole of the medical school hierarchy should attend. It rapidly gained status and each year the main lecture theatre would be packed. With all this interest the students became more and more imaginative with their presentations until ultimately they became stage presentations with music, lights, projections and costumes, replacing the boring old overhead transparencies. About 9 or 10 years ago I was interviewing candidates for a new consultant post in surgery for a hospital in Kent. One of the candidates include in his CV, "winner of the Golden Finger Award" Cardiff 1986. Naturally he got the job but I hope my legacy will amount to more than that.

Sadly, with the modernisation of the teaching curriculum, the surgical teaching firm has all but disappeared, a great loss in my opinion.

During my time in Cardiff I embarked on two very important strands of research. One was linked to the measurement of a patient's quality of life (QOL), and the other concerned the use of tamoxifen. My interest here was contingent on my partnership with Dr. Terry Priestman, an oncologist who worked at the Velindre cancer hospital. Every week we did a combined clinic to look after the needs of the women with advanced breast cancer.

We were amongst the very first to use tamoxifen (known by its commercial name Nolvadex [ICI 46,474] in those days). Dr. Arthur Walpole PhD discovered Tamoxifen in 1966 whilst on a drug discovery programme for contraceptive agents on behalf of ICI. (Figure 34)

It was indeed an anti-oestrogen but also had a paradoxical effect of provoking ovulation and acting as a fertility drug. Much lab based work by Craig Jordan in Shrewsbury, Mass. USA, Rob Nicholson at the Tenovus institute in Cardiff, and Mitch Dowsett at the Royal Marsden London, ultimately explained this paradox and provided a safe theoretical base for future clinical studies; but it was Mary Cole in 1971 who, following a leap of intuition, used it first in clinical cases of advanced breast cancer. Terry and I started using it in 1972/3 and were surprised at its low toxicity and efficacy. The drug produced durable remissions in about 30% of cases, with few side effects. This

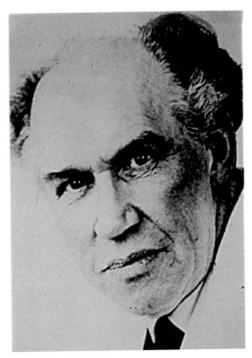

Fig. 34 Dr. Arthur Walpole

persuaded us to launch a clinical trial comparing tamoxifen with conventional chemotherapy in cases of advanced breast cancer. At this point it is worth remembering, as described in the preface to this book, the tragic circumstances of my mother's terminal illness. With this in the back of my mind I thought it might be a good idea if, as well as objective response rates and length of survival, we also factored in subjective outcomes to measure QOL. As none existed at the time we had to invent one. The inspiration for this came from an advert for some proprietary potion that would improve your sense of well being if you felt "one degree under".

If you could feel one degree under then 100 degrees might mean you felt perfect so what was wanted was a thermometer that measured feelings rather than temperature. This lead to the birth of the first psychometric instrument for measuring QOL that we christened LASA, standing for Linear Analogue Self Assessment. Their were 25 domains represented by a line each measuring 100mm. The ends of the line marked the extremes with 100 as "never felt better" and 0 as close to death. These domains included pain, depression, anxiety, physical activity, sexual activity and a rounded up score for "well being". The patient acted as their own control and added crosses along the lines of LASA and we simply measured the outcomes in millimetres comparing outcomes on treatment with QOL at baseline. The measures seemed to reflect what was going on and even seemed to give early notice of a poor outcome with the LASA scores falling before objective measures of progression became apparent. I remember with painful clarity the first time I presented these data. It was at a meeting sponsored by ICI and in those days there was no limit to the hospitality that could be provided by a pharmaceutical company. The evening before my presentation we were treated to a banquet that involved 7 different wines and a brandy nightcap. I woke up the next morning feeling great without realizing I was still inebriated. I gave a brilliant talk fuelled by the Chateau Yquem and Remy Martin of the night before. After my talk a questioner from the floor, looking puzzled, asked me how we measured sexual satisfaction. I replied; "it's easy, we do it in millimetres". This provoked gales of laughter and I had to go and lie down with a splitting headache. Nevertheless our work was appreciated and the Lancet published our paper on LASA whilst the BMJ published two papers on the direct comparison of Nolvadex with chemotherapy. In the first paper we showed that chemotherapy produced earlier and greater objective remissions whilst in the second paper we showed that in the longer term the survival was the same, but Nolvadex was associated with a better QOL. John Forbes was a co-author of these papers and on his return to Australia repeated these studies on a much larger scale through the ANZ group, confirming our original findings. However there was an important variable missing from our trials and that was knowledge of the oestrogen receptor status of the tumours (ER).

Before I explain the nature and importance of the ER a short digression is in order.

In 1893 George Beatson was appointed consulting surgeon to the Glasgow Cancer Hospital, and from then on he was dedicated to the search for better methods of diagnosis and treatment of cancer in women. In 1896 he published in The Lancet his famous paper, 'The Treatment of Inoperable Cases of Carcinoma of the Mamma: Suggestions for a New Method of Treatment with Illustrative Cases'. His earlier studies on the effect of ovarian function on lactation in cows had 'pointed to one organ holding control over the secretion of another and separate organ'. Observing also that 'the changes that take place in the mammary gland in the process of lactation are almost identical, up to a certain point, with what takes place in a cancerous mamma', he became the first surgeon ever to remove the ovaries from women with inoperable breast cancer. His paper recounted the case histories of three such operations that he had performed in 1895. His patients were not cured, but the marked improvement in local lesions that he reported in the 1896 Lancet article encouraged others to follow up his work, and this eventually led to the modern use of endocrine therapy in breast cancer.

However a more recent study of Beatson's operating log carried out by David Smith, a distinguished Scottish surgeon, pointed out that Beatson had in fact carried out 9 such procedures but only reported his successes. This one out of three ratio for response to endocrine therapy in advanced breast cancer continued to apply irrespective of whether the intervention was ovarian castration, adrenalectomy or removal of the pituitary gland, not to mention Nolvadex the first oral endocrine therapy. It wasn't until Ellwood Jensen, (Figure 35) whose original work in the 1950s in Chicago predicted a specific oestrogen binding protein in hormone responsive tissues, that some sense was made of this magic one in three ratio.

By the late 1970s assays were becoming available for human tissue to determine whether or not they carried the ER and at the same time separated breast cancers into two groups ER+ and ER–. The former were the ones that responded and the latter the ones that had acquired

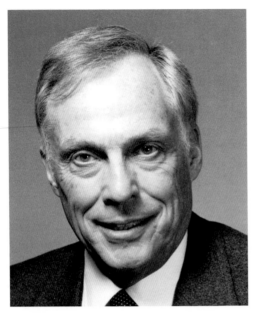

Fig. 35 Dr. Ellwood Jensen

resistance. Today using relatively simple staining techniques with the monoclonal antibody to the ER, it has become a routine service to classify breast cancers in these two groups in order to offer targeted therapy. Such tests were not available in the mid 1970s so we went about it on the "suck it and see" principle. This was alright for a tablet like Nolvadex but a cruel gamble when trying out castration or the frightful operations required to remove both adrenal glands that perch on top of the kidneys or the pituitary gland hidden at the base of the brain awfully close to the nerves responsible for vision. Mind you, sucking a tamoxifen tablet is no joke either as I once found to my cost. I was trying to persuade a non-English speaking member of the royal family of a Middle Eastern Sultanate that she starts on the medicine. In response to her sceptical body language I popped a pill in my mouth and found it too large to swallow, so I chewed it up. I cannot describe the foul metallic taste that blasted my taste buds but gamely I kept on smiling, leaving the room in a hurry to lie with my mouth under a tap.

The taste remained with me for 24 hours and was only relieved by 50 millilitres of an 18-year-old Talisker the following evening.

Based on my experience in using tamoxifen in advanced breast cancer and the increasing interest in the biological mechanisms of response involved in hormone therapy for cancer, I wrote a paper advocating adjuvant tamoxifen in the management of the early disease. Now, as I described earlier, the therapeutic consequence of the Fisherian model of breast cancer that envisaged the disease as systemic i.e. widespread at the point of diagnosis, was the belief that some form of "adjuvant" systemic therapy targeting these putative but occult micro-metastases might favourably influence the natural history of the disease. At the same time Bernie Fisher's group in the USA and Gianni Bonadonna in Milan were embarking on the first trials of adjuvant chemotherapy. I argued that tamoxifen would be less toxic but at the same time might only be relevant in about 30% of cases.

Shortly after this paper appeared I was visited by the young doctor John Patterson, an up-and-coming clinical scientist working for ICI. In short he suggested putting money where my mouth was. (John went on to become a member of the triumvirate at the very top of the management pyramid of Astra Zeneca.) We then went about putting together a multicentre clinical trial steering committee, developing a protocol and raising the funding. The first of these tasks was aided by the fact that Professor Sir Patrick Forrest, (Figure 36) the Regius professor of surgery in Edinburgh, had just established the first specialist group in Europe for those interested in breast cancer. Initially this was called the British Breast Club but after

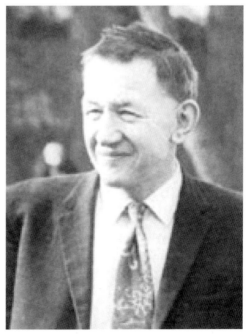

Fig. 36 Professor Sir Patrick Forrest

some confusion with a double booking with an organization with the same initials, it became the British Breast Group (BBG). The BBG started off more as a dining club with the two main criteria for membership being an interest in the disease and that intangible British characteristic of "clubbability". As a result our meetings were riotous and great fun, yet the sense of mutual respect and affection demonstrated again by the British mannerism of loudly insulting your best friends whilst being steely polite to your enemies, lead to the most fruitful and exciting academic debates I've ever experienced. The BBG without a doubt placed the subject on the map, successfully demanded sufficient resources from the NHS and acted as a template for future sub-specialization in medicine and surgery.

Having got my steering committee together we had to start developing a protocol, but the first step was to dream up a catchy acronym for the trial. I can't remember who came up with the title but we eventually decided on Nolvadex Adjuvant Trial Organization or NATO for short. This time we hoped that the Americans would be sufficiently confused by the name as to read our publications. The point being that Americans in spite of all their virtues remain solipsist in their global view and if the work wasn't carried out in the States it might go unnoticed.

The design of the trial was simple: any woman eligible for surgery for early breast cancer was randomized to take 20 mgm of tamoxifen a day for two years or to act as a control with tamoxifen in reserve in case of relapse. (I've often been asked why we elected to prescribe it for two years; blowed if I can remember, it just seemed a good idea at the time and we got lucky.) We also decided to test a "second order hypothesis" to see if the benefit, if any, was to be sequestrated to those women bearing ER+ tumours. This latter ambition was a great challenge as the assay was difficult with only a few laboratories tooled up to carry it out. In the end we settled on a central lab facility at the ICRF in Lincoln's Inn Fields, London. Unfortunately that meant the rapid freezing of samples in liquid nitrogen at the time of surgery and transporting them by train in thermos flasks packed in insulated boxes. One delivery to Paddington was X-rayed and found to contain a metallic cylinder, suspected of being a bomb, and detonated on the platform by security staff at the time of intense IRA activity in the capital. In the end ICI and the Cancer Research Campaign (CRC) funded the whole project jointly.

The first patient was recruited in 1977 and 1,200 patients entered the study by 1979.

Our first results were published in The Lancet in 1983 and I remember thinking they were too good to be true as they showed a 30% relative risk reduction for relapse amongst those taking the drug. Disappointing in retrospect was our failure to demonstrate that the ER status of the tumour had predictive value for response. For some years afterwards I argued that tamoxifen mediated its response via another mechanism independent of the ER content of the tumour but I was ultimately silenced when the 1990 overview of all the tamoxifen trials confirmed that the ER status was a powerful predictor of response. I have little doubt now that the assay we were using was faulty and many of the specimens were incorrectly labelled as ER – because the protein decayed in transit and at least one was detonated in Paddington station at the height of "the troubles" in Northern Ireland.

A year or two before this milestone publication Fisher's group (NSABP) and Bonadonna's group in Italy had reported very promising early results from adjuvant combination chemotherapy. The stage was then set for a battle between the hawks and the doves that raged for 15 years, and was finally settled when further trials suggested that both groups had a share in the truth. A combination of both approaches, if the patient's tumour was ER+, could improve relapse-free survival by about 50%. From a peak in 1985 breast cancer mortality in the UK for both pre and postmenopausal women started falling rapidly and about half that benefit could be attributed to tamoxifen. (Figure 37)

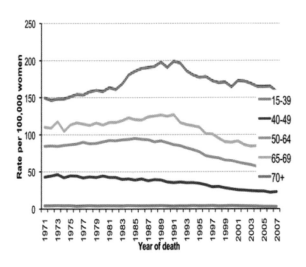

Fig. 37 Trends in breast cancer mortality since the introduction of adjuvant systemic therapy

Chapter 9

King's again 1979–1989

In 1979 I was appointed to the chair of surgery at King's College London, but located on the campus of the hospital and medical school at King's College Hospital, Denmark Hill. I was to replace my old chief Professor Murray who was shortly to retire and was appointed over the head of the then reader in surgery, my old friend and mentor Colin Howe. He never showed any animosity and welcomed me with open arms. However before I settled in to my clinical and academic challenges, I had the more immediate challenges of finding somewhere to live and somewhere to send my kids to school. The differential in house prices between London and Cardiff had if anything widened over the previous seven years. I couldn't even afford to buy back my little box in Forest Hill. After much house hunting and soul searching, we settled on an old Victorian vicarage that had seen better days in a road that had seen better inhabitants in an unfashionable area of East Dulwich within easy reach of the hospital. The house had some antique charm and there was an old walled garden but some of the neighbours were delinquent problem families who had been re-housed by the council. Even so I could barely keep up the mortgage repayments and that was before school fees.

Against all my socialist principles and against all the advice of my bank manager, we entered Richard into Dulwich College, a famous and ancient public school. He hated it, but the alternative was the local blackboard jungle that kept the local delinquent children off the street until they were 16. These kids, as represented by some of our near neighbours, graduated from petty crime to major league gangsterism within 5 years, bypassing the need for any O levels. I hate to catch myself writing this self-justification but those were the realities of the choices we faced. In truth the state school he would have attended, because of our catchment area, was later closed down because of the uncontrolled violence and crime amongst the schoolboys. Katie and Suzanne at least were offered the safe haven of the local Church of England primary school, although I could imagine the fury of my late paternal grandfather had he witnessed them reciting The Lord's Prayer off by heart and singing, "All things bright and beautiful". Needs must....

After a couple more years, when Judy could no longer bear being spat at and cursed by the neighbourhood children, we decamped to a less attractive house with a much larger mortgage in the safer and prettier area of Dulwich village.

Even so the house appeared to be mysteriously empty and underpriced and it took some time before I discovered it had belonged to a member of the notorious South London Richardson gang. The owner was wanted for murder and was hiding somewhere on the Costa Brava and the mysterious holes in the lawn were lasting evidence of the futile efforts of the Metropolitan Police to find the missing body. Well at least that's one way of providing affordable housing for health workers.

I had three problems to confront on taking over the chair at King's. The first was that I had inherited a top-heavy department. In addition to Colin Howe, reader in surgery and my official deputy, there were two other professors with personal chairs who had come up through the ranks. Although I held the established chair and head of department, my two old friends and colleagues, Vijay Kakkar and Alan Bennett, had been promoted in my absence from lecturer, to senior lecturer and then to a professorship on the merit of their published work. Vijay was a tall and handsome Indian, a look alike for Omar Sharif, who had joined the department as a lowly research fellow at the same time as me in 1965. He had taken on the challenge of thrombosis and surgery and his brilliant research has since saved thousands of deaths from pulmonary embolism all round the world. We bonded in the first week of meeting and share a warm sense of mutual respect to this day. His son Ajay has followed in his footsteps and is now professor of surgery at Bart's. Vijay and his wife invited Judy and me for an "Indian evening" shortly after we met. We started off in a curry house and then went on to see Oh Calcutta! Vijay and his wife Savi didn't know where to look when it became apparent that the show was far from Indian, but was in fact the rudest and nudest musical ever staged in London.

Alan Bennett was a brilliant pharmacologist working in the department's laboratories, having been recruited by professor Murray to study the physiology and pharmacology of gastric acid secretion. His work on prostaglandins was ground breaking. We had a lot in common and together with his wife Rochelle and our youngest children went away together for vacations. He played a mean tenor sax and a mean game of squash. Sadly he died a few years ago of prostate cancer, one of the diseases he was researching upon. The upshot of this was that although I was chairman of the department I had no one to share my workload.

The corollary to this was my next problem of having to raise my own money to appoint staff to assist in my line of research. The third problem was that whilst Vijay and Allan had been building their empires, the old department had become almost moribund.

However I did have one advantage and that was the fact that I still remained chairman of the clinical trials group with a portfolio of two trials, the first King's/Cambridge study and the NATO trial. On the strength of this I went to the CRC with the ambitious proposal for a purpose-built clinical trials centre, the first in Europe, to house the staff of these two studies and to provide a professional infrastructure for national cancer trials in the future. This was based upon my experience in working in the NSABP office in Pittsburgh. To my delight and amazement they agreed.

With this injection of cash and some additional wheeling and dealing with the medical school, I was able to build myself a nice new department with a nice new office befitting my status. My office enjoyed rosewood furniture and bookcases with the nice finishing touch of a high backed, leather upholstered, swivel chair. All this was achieved within a year of me taking office, but I was not to take possession of the chair until the CRC had organized an official opening ceremony and that was contingent on the availability of Lady Cavendish, the CRC's honorary president. That was to be the 1st of September, two weeks or so after Richard's bar-mitzvah celebrations. That in itself was not a problem, but I was committed to a lecture tour as a visiting professor in New Zealand that would make it a close call. Then to add to my problems the rabbi found he had double booked the Sabbath in question so the celebration was shifted a week later leaving me precisely eight days to fly around the world giving lectures in Auckland, Christchurch and Dunedin. Judy said I was mad and should cancel but I hated to let people down and considered myself superman.

Bar-mitzvahs in my community are big deals. As a rite of passage it's a cross between a coming of age and first communion and an opportunity for the young man to show off his Hebrew scholarship and singing voice in the synagogue. It is also the first opportunity for the young man's father to show off his wealth. As I had no wealth at this time I entered into the phase of what is now known as negative equity, by taking out a second mortgage. Anyway we had a lovely party in a big marquee in the garden, Richard made us proud and I was provided with my first chance of delivering a long, boring and self indulgent speech, on the basis that as I was paying for dinner then I had paid for my guests to shut up and listen.

The following morning, to Judy's intense displeasure, I flew off in a westerly direction en route to Auckland. That's about as far as you can go before meeting yourself coming back. The last but one of the legs of this journey was between LA and Tahiti. On landing in this tropical paradise we were hit by a tropical storm that left me stranded in the transit lounge for 24 hours. I arrived in Auckland on the evening of my first lecture and was rushed straight to the hall in the same clothes I'd been wearing for 48 hours, not knowing what day or what hour it was. As I'd crossed a date line it was something like breakfast time the day before yesterday. I delivered my lecture on autopilot and crashed out. The following morning I awoke in the middle of the night and realized that what with the celebrations at home and the long flight, I hadn't had my bowels open for nearly 5 days. Unfortunately my gastrointestinal tract had gone to sleep or was suffering from terminal jet lag. The net result sparing you a few unnecessary details was that I developed prolapsed thrombosed piles.

My next lecture in Christchurch was delivered in agony whilst I tried to achieve some temporary comfort by discretely sitting on the tip of the billiard cue I was using as a pointer. That evening I was to dine with the host faculty in the house of the chief of surgery, the delightful professor Shackleton.

Before dinner I told him of my plight. He then took me to his consulting rooms attached to his house and provided me with both topical and systemic analgesics. On entering the dining room I noticed that his thoughtful wife had provided *everybody* with an additional cushion to sit on so as not to draw attention to my embarrassing malaise. This was but the first example of the wonderful kindness I have experienced jet setting round the world as a visiting professor. I managed to complete my tour and returned home utterly exhausted, totally spaced out and in absolute agony, just in time for the next ordeal in presiding over the official opening of my department. Even when that was over I still couldn't occupy my chair in my new office, in fact I couldn't occupy any kind of chair at that time; so I admitted myself as an emergency to the Royal London hospital under a pseudonym, for the attention of the king of perineal surgery, the top man at the bottom end, the inventor of "Parks' painless pilectomy", the peerless Sir Alan Parks.

Painless it was not, yet out of this adversity I learnt many lessons. Firstly patients are treated in a patronizing way and forced to wear pyjamas day and night for no other reason than matron's convenience. Secondly post-operative analgesia is given too little too late, and thirdly that I was not superhuman and should in future listen to the words of wisdom of my wife from time to time.

At long last I was able to settle into my chair. First of all I had to recruit some staff. A key to a happy professor is to have a diligent senior lecturer to delegate clinical, teaching and administrative work. Unfortunately as explained, the established posts were filled by personal professors so I had to make do with a lowly lecturer instead. Along the way I enjoyed the company of many talented young men and women who I mentored, all of whom went on to great things either in the academic or NHS sectors.

I then raised the funds for the first clinical nurse specialist to train up as a counsellor. The role was taken by Sister Sylvia Denton OBE, who went on to found this new discipline and ended up as president of the Royal College of Nursing. Next I appointed Joan Houghton to become my first professional data manager/clinical trials coordinator. She was promoted as the staff levels grew to become the manager of the clinical trials centre. Joan invented many of the systems in place for running RCTS all round the world to this day. Finally I appointed Lesley Fallowfield to start up a new section in my department on "psycho-social" oncology. Her task was to carry forward my earlier work on QOL and to start teaching communication skills. Lesley is now professor of psychosocial oncology at the University of Sussex having virtually invented the subject from scratch. She also runs a national course for teaching senior oncologists, consultants, senior lecturers and professors the art of good communication with patients. Even I have not been spared the ritual humiliation of exposing my limitations in communication skills in the presence of my peers.

We now have an International society for psychosocial oncology (ISOQOL) that has given me much pride and further excuses for a bit of onco-tourism to glamorous parts of the world.

I wish to put that aside for the moment and describe the mature results of the King's/Cambridge trial (CRC 1) and the NATO trial that had provided the raison d'être for the CRC trials centre in the first place. By the time I got back to King's in 1980 CRC 1 had recruited over 3,000 patients and as it matured over the next few years a pattern began to appear. Professor Jack Cuzick who was leading statistical consultant to the department drew this trend to my attention. He noted a quite uncanny difference in outcome between right sided and left sided breast cancers. Although overall there was no difference in 10-year survival whether or not the women had radiotherapy, there appeared to be a qualitative difference between left and right. Women with left-sided cancers were more likely to die of heart disease and less likely to die of breast cancer if they had postoperative radiotherapy and vice versa in the absence of radiotherapy. Although judged implausible at the time a closer look at the data suggested that irradiating the left breast using the techniques of the day damaged the coronary arteries just below the rib cage leading to an excess of heart attacks. I remember the first time I delivered a talk on this subject at the joint centre for radiotherapy in the Dana Farber Institute Boston Mass; I was greeted not only with scepticism but outright hostility. In the fullness of time our results were acknowledged and replicated in other studies as a consequence of which techniques were modified in order to avoid the left anterior descending coronary artery. Without a large scale RCT this subtle effect would have been overlooked. Today the latest results comparing surgery to the breast with and without radiotherapy have confirmed an important 5–7% improvement in survival now that the effect is no longer diluted out by an excess of deaths from non-cancer causes.

As far as the NATO trial was concerned as already described we published the first results in the Lancet in 1983 but the real breakthrough for adjuvant tamoxifen came a couple of years later in 1985 with the first world "overview" analysis. The seeds for this were sown after a meeting in my office in 1984 when Richard Peto came to call. Richard, now Professor Sir Richard Peto, is Professor of Medical Statistics & Epidemiology at the University of Oxford. He is without doubt one of the leading intellectuals of the age and has made major contributions to the eradication of tobacco and the fall in cancer mortality throughout the world. In 1984 his shock of blond hair that fell across his eyes and his excitable demeanour gave him the appearance of a boy band rock star on speed. The hair is now grey but the speed is still apparent.

Almost incoherent with excitement he showed me the first printout of a meta-analysis of all the data of all the extant trials of adjuvant tamoxifen, published or unpublished, from around the world. The fact that he had got hold of the data was a tribute to his art of persuasion and the method of the analysis was a tribute to his mathematical genius. Without bothering you with the details of the maths, an overview or meta-analysis is a statistically valid way of summating the results from many trials of similar design that avoids publication bias and weights the results according to the power (sample size) of each of the studies included. Prominent among the other trials were studies from Scotland and Sweden as well as CRC2 that we started up after NATO had completed accrual. The data Richard showed me demonstrated beyond a shadow of doubt that at last we had something relatively non- toxic, that could reduce breast cancer mortality by a substantial amount. Richard and his team in Oxford then set about organizing the first world overview of what we christened the Early Breast Cancer Trials Collaborative Group (EBCTCG) that took place in 1985. That meeting proved a seminal event in the history of breast cancer and also demonstrated that chemotherapy had a dramatic effect, although at first that seemed to be confined to the premenopausal women. From that date, when we were witnessing a peak in breast cancer mortality in the UK, there has been a fall in breast cancer deaths of close on 50% in both pre and post-menopausal women, as clinicians almost overnight adopted one or other form of adjuvant systemic therapy. Every 5 years the EBCTCG meets in Oxford and each time the outcomes seem to get better with each incremental improvement in the design and selection criteria for the treatments. This international collaboration shows science working at it's best for man/womankind and I feel very proud to have taken a role in the proceedings, although Richard Peto deserves all the credit for his inexhaustible energy and enthusiasm, not forgetting his mathematical genius. In the same way that the invention of the microscope by Anton van Leeuwenhoek in the early 17thC allowed us to see what was hidden in the microcosm of the cell so in my mind the invention of the meta-analysis has allowed us to see with beautiful clarity what is hidden in the macrocosm of large numbers.

Whilst all this was going on Jack Cuzick made another chance finding in our tamoxifen database. It appeared that those patients randomized to receive tamoxifen had only half the chance of developing contralateral disease (i.e. a new cancer in the other breast that is not a recurrence of the initial primary tumour). From this observation that was also confirmed in the overview together with laboratory studies by Craig Jordan and pioneering work by Trevor Powles of the Royal Marsden, the scene was set for the race to discover a chemical way to prevent the disease in the first place, but I'll leave it to others to tell that tale.

Chapter 10

Trials and Tribulations

"It is not truisms that science unveils. Rather, it is part of the greatness and the beauty of science that we can learn, through our own critical investigations, that the world is utterly different from what we ever imagined –"

Karl Popper

I had always been interested in the history and philosophy of science since embarking on my academic career in the early 1970s. This was in part due to the influence of my brother, Professor Harold Baum, who went on to become Dean of Life Science at King's College, London. He was the one that taught me Baum's theorem that all odd numbers are prime.

One is odd and prime, three is odd and prime, five is odd and prime, seven is odd and prime, nine is an experimental error, eleven is odd and prime, thirteen is odd and prime Q.E.D.

I even went so far as to list this interest, along with the history of fine art amongst the subjects I dabbled in, when composing my first entry into Who's Who. I identified myself as a "Popperian" for reasons of taxonomy and a wish to impress my friends. You can therefore imagine my surprised delight on hearing from my hero in person sometime in 1991, when I was invited to look after a close friend of Karl who had just been diagnosed with breast cancer. When I asked him "why me?" he replied that it was because of my entry in Who's Who. (Figure 38)

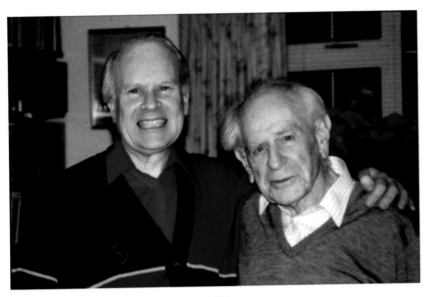

Fig. 38 Karl Popper and me, circa 1992

If I wanted a surgeon to cut me open my first wish would be that he was a master of his craft, the fact that he might have an interest in philosophy would be well down on the list of personal traits I would be looking for.

Nevertheless things went well and I became pretty friendly with the old man in the last few years of his life. We exchanged letters on matters philosophical and I was invited to tea on the very day he took delivery of the first Russian translation of "The Open Society and its Enemies". In his excitement he signed a copy of the English version for me, which remains one of my most precious keepsakes. The last communication I had from Karl was a letter dated 4/1/93, referring to some papers I sent for him to critique, upon which he commented favourably. The last line of his last letter read; "For me, the most interesting of your papers was, 'Limitations of non-science in Surgical Epistemology', I hope you may find time, one day, to discuss these issues with me." Sadly I didn't.

There is an old joke doing the rounds of the cocktail party circuit that runs as follows: A hostess introduces two strangers to each other, one a doctor and the other a lawyer. The lawyer goes on to say 'Oh so you're a doctor. I must tell you this screamingly funny story about a surgeon'. To which the doctor replies 'I think before you go any further, I ought to warn you that I am a surgeon'. Quick as a flash the lawyer responds: 'in which case I will tell it very slowly!' Once again the stereotype of the surgeon is reinforced as an unthinking technician, so the idea of a 'philosophical surgeon' might be read as an oxymoron.

In defence of the thinking surgeon, I wish to propose that a modern surgeon practising evidence-based, humane and ethical medicine, must have a sound grounding in some of the fundamental principles of philosophy.

The epistemology of medicine

Epistemology is a bit of a mouthful that simply means the study or the theory of the growth of knowledge – or putting it another way, how is it that we know certain facts to be true. At the most simple level our observations can be misleading, and so called 'common sense' is no substitute for a systematic approach to the acquisition of knowledge. Primitive man 'knew' that the Earth was flat and that the Earth was the centre of the universe. For all intents and purposes it made little difference to the way of life in primitive communities, but these firmly held beliefs were false. The recognition that the world was round and that the universe was heliocentric rather than geocentric were scientific observations of seismic importance in the history of mankind.

All undergraduates should understand this period of history where the theories of Copernicus and the observations of Galileo changed man's status in the universe, and opened minds to a systematic pursuit of knowledge from the age of enlightenment to the present day. The playwright Bertold Brecht put the following words into the mouth of Galileo: 'It is not the purpose of our science to open the gates to infinite wisdom but merely to set the limits to the extent of our ignorance.' If that is indeed the case for the study of cosmology, which has little impact on the day-to-day life of even the most sophisticated communities, how much more so does it apply to our lives when facing their premature end under the threat of cancer or cardiovascular disease?

It was Aristotle and other great names of the golden age of Pericles in the ancient city of Athens who were the first to apply a systematic approach to the pursuit of knowledge. They recognised that our conceptual model of the world around us was a figment of our imagination, and it was therefore necessary to systematically collect observations to challenge this view. These observations were built up into a conceptual model (hypothesis), and later observations were selected to corroborate this model.

The process of collecting observations in defence of a hypothesis is known as inductivism. Inductive logic was considered 'science' up until the eighteenth century, when the Scottish philosopher David Hume finally illustrated the poverty of the process. Perhaps the best way of illustrating the poverty of inductivism as it relates to our lives as medical practitioners is to consider the subject of *alternative medicine*.

When doctors attack alternative medicine or appear sceptical to its much-trumpeted claims, we are often accused of being bigots with closed minds, protecting a closed shop. Nothing could be further from the truth, but it has taken a layman, the late great John Diamond, to find the words to set the record straight. For that reason I would like to quote from his posthumously published book 'Snake Oil and other Preoccupations'.

'I am not an academic and this is not an academic book, even though the facts I list in it have a perfectly good scientific basis to them but when it comes to human motivation I am working blind. I can only guess why most people seem to prefer the unproven to the proven, the anecdotal to the rigorously demonstrated, and the so-called natural to the scientific'.

There is much within that passage, on the nature of proof, the nature of the scientific method, and the use and abuse of anecdotal evidence.

The alternative practitioner can trace his roots back to Galen in the second century, and a metaphysical belief system based on the balance of *natural humours*. For example, Galen believed that breast cancer was due to an excess of *black bile* (melancholia). Inductive support for this belief came from the observation that breast cancer was more common in post-menopausal women than pre-menopausal women, and this was thought to be because the menstrual flux in pre-menopausal women got rid of the putative excess of black bile. The therapeutic consequences of this belief therefore were purgation and venesection (bloodletting). The inductive 'proof' that this approach worked were the anecdotes about women with breast cancer who were treated by purgation and venesection, and who lived for several years after diagnosis. Those who died were the victims of the bloodletter who didn't have the courage of his convictions, or the patient herself who lacked the constitutional vigour to sustain prolonged bloodletting.

There is a neo-Galenic doctrine, based on the view that breast cancer is indeed due to an imbalance of nature, only substituting *energy fields* for the natural humours. According to this view, to restore perfect health you have to restore the balance of these metaphysical *energy fields*. This might be achieved by acupuncture balancing out the ying and the yang, homeopathy (*similia similibus curentur*), or strange balancing diets. The Gerson diet in particular is very fashionable.

In fact, one of my patients, seeking to improve my education, gave me a book describing this approach. The first half of the book formulated the hypothesis why this strange diet should improve the balance of the immune system, and the second half of the book consisted of 50 anecdotes of patients with cancer, who were only given six months to live by the medical profession, took the diet and lived for a long time.

The trouble with that kind of evidence is that although we know the numerator (50) we don't know the denominator – for example, 50 out of 1000 cases treated by neglect could indeed live for many years while the indolent disease progresses on the chest wall. Furthermore, from the evidence available in the book some of the diagnoses were a little bit shaky and the author neglects to mention whether or not these patients received conventional treatment at the same time as the magic diet. Finally, I know of no oncologist who gives a patient six months to live. We may say that the median survival for a group with advanced cancer is six months, but among this group certain individuals may lie at extremes of survival. These individuals are the substance of the anecdote.

I once rather mischievously tried to illustrate this in a paper I wrote for "World Medicine" in 1982. It was entitled "Sensory deprivation project (SDP)" and coincided with the launch of the new political party the Social Democrats, also known as SDP. I argued that stress in the modern environment was the cause of cancer because the never ending assault on our sensory systems raised our plasma cortisol levels. It was a "well known fact" that cortisone depressed the immune system and it was also a "well known fact" that the immune system protected against cancer. It followed therefore that a period of sensory deprivation would be good for cancer. I then described a fictitious unit where cancer patients were locked up in a dark and silent room and fed intravenously for six months. I made up a series of 20 patients who had only been given six months to live. 10 died before they completed their treatment; pity they weren't referred earlier. 5 dropped out the programme so could be discounted, but 5 completed the programme and lived on for another 6 to 12 months. In case anyone had missed the point I ended by requesting donations to support the SDP.

Well, as you've probably guessed by now, I had patients referred by GPs for SDP and received donations for my wonderful research! I was mortified and returned the donations and explained the spoof to a number of furious patients and doctors before writing an abject apology in the next issue of the journal.

Perhaps I should leave the last word on this subject by quoting from Robert Parks' wonderful book *Voodoo Science*.

'Alternative seems to define a culture rather than a field of medicine – a culture that is not scientifically demanding. It is a culture in which ancient accretions are given more weight than biological science and anecdotes are preferred over clinical trials. Alternative therapies steadfastly resist change often for centuries or even millennia, unaffected by scientific advances in the understanding of physiology or disease'.

If that is the case then who are the bigots and who are the ones with the closed minds?

The alternative to alternative medicine should be scientific medicine, not 'orthodoxy'. By science, I mean the application of deductive logic. The deductive approach starts with the formulation of the hypothesis, but for a start the hypothesis must be rational in its explanation of the disease process or therapeutic intervention. By 'rational' I mean built upon the growth of knowledge of human biology and physiology from the past 100 years or so, without invoking magic or metaphysical principles.

Even so, the new hypothesis is still perceived as a fictional account of reality and subjected to rigorous test by the design of experiments challenging the new theory with the 'hazard of refutation'. These experiments in medical or surgical therapeutics must have control groups treated by observation, placebo or 'best available therapy'. Without the control group we merely have a series of anecdotal reports. What I have just described is in fact a randomised controlled trial.

Let me tell you a little story that illustrates the advantage of deductive over inductive logic that for the most part is true.

When my youngest daughter Suzanne was about 4 years old we had a black cat with the misnomer of Lucky. Lucky was loved and tormented in equal measure. One dark evening it ran across the road only to be flattened by a passing truck. Sue was inconsolable and we offered her a replacement. After sober thought she said yes please but can it be a white cat. "Why a white cat?" I asked. "It's 'cause white cats is easier to see on the road at night than black cats" she replied. An interesting hypothesis for a 4 year old I thought. Eventually a neighbour gave us a white kitten from the litter of her own moggie. The kitten grew into a somewhat indolent cat and one day when my wife was vacuum cleaning the carpet around the sleeping cat she reached the conclusion that the cat was deaf. I investigated that claim and concluded that the puss was indeed deaf and together with the pink eyes was probably an albino. That cat also reached a sticky end under the wheels of the number 27 bus on Lordship Lane. Looking up the mortality statistics on cats in SE London I noted that black cats had three times the rate of death from road traffic accidents than white cats proving that my daughter's hypothesis was true. But wait, that is an inductive proof. On closer inspection of the data I noted that white albino cats were rare mutants and were twelve times less common than the black phenotype. Redoing the stats using *chi squared analysis* (trust me on this one) I could demonstrate that the Sue-by-hypothesis had been falsified and that white cats had a significant disadvantage on the roads at night probably because they can't hear the number 27 bus approaching.

Making use of these new data I might even have been able to protect albino cats by providing them with hearing aids marketed as "felinofones".

Anyway let's get back to breast cancer before the men in white coats come to take me away.

In the late 1970s and early 1980s the treatment of patients within clinical trials was the exception rather than the rule. I take some grim satisfaction that the opposite applies today even to the point that the percent of patients entered into a RCT is now considered a quality outcome measure in specialist cancer centres. However 20 or 30 years ago many of the profession and most lay people, if they thought about clinical trials at all, considered them "human experimentation" and, for treatment to be decided at the toss of a coin, totally unacceptable. The best way to illustrate this is for me to describe the decline and fall of the CRC breast conservation trial that in part contributed to my own decline and fall.

Preservation of the breast in the treatment of breast cancer was not a new idea in the 1980s. Sir Geoffrey Keynes, senior surgeon at Bart's, published a paper on this in the BMJ in 1937. This was illustrated with a beautiful anatomical line drawing showing the positioning of radium needles in the retained breast following "lumpectomy". (Figure 28 on p. 67) It is worth noting that the placement of the radioactive needles includes the whole of the retained breast tissue as well as all the regional lymphatic fields. So although the outcome was conservative the intention was radical and therefore another expression of the orthodox paradigm. The fact that his results looked favourable might simply have been due to bias in his selection of case material. That aside his approach was not accepted with any enthusiasm and in his autobiography, "The Gates of Memory", published at the age of 94, Keynes describes the hostility he met from the profession even to the point that his lectures were boycotted on a visit to the USA. Unfortunately the storm clouds of war were gathering over Europe and Keynes was busy setting up the first blood transfusion service in the UK. At the outbreak of the Second World War Keynes was called up to act as head of the RAF medical corps. When Bart's had a near miss during the London blitz, Keynes' radium needles were buried for safety and along with that the debate about breast conserving surgery was buried for the next 40 years. The subject was reopened by George Crile, a distinguished and open minded surgeon at the Cleveland clinic in the early 1970s, although he never carried out a formal trial, and a little later by Bernard Fisher who had the courage to launch a RCT. In a television debate with Gerry Urban from the Memorial Sloane Kettering Institute in New York, the leading proponent of super radical mastectomy of the time, Fisher was accused of unethical behaviour not by virtue of advocating a RCT but by daring to challenge the prevailing orthodoxy.

Sir Hedley Atkins and John Hayward at Guy's Hospital London launched a small RCT comparing radical mastectomy with lumpectomy (an ugly term) plus radiotherapy. The conduct of the trial was flawed and it gave rather misleading results suggesting that the radical procedure was superior. In the end it was the trials by Umberto Veronesi in Milan and Fisher's NSABP trial in the USA that eventually settled the matter. Umberto Veronesi was a tall, handsome and flamboyant Italian of noble ancestry. In many ways he pioneered the techniques of breast preservation and his Istituto dei Tumori in Milan became legendary, as it was also the home of Gianni Bonadonna, one of the pioneers of adjuvant chemotherapy. Veronesi eventually became minister of health in Italy but gave that up when he established the European Institute of Cancer. There is no doubt that Fisher and Veronesi were the two pillars of surgical oncology in the world at the time, bestriding the Atlantic like twin colossi.

Trying to emulate these two great men I was responsible for launching the CRC breast conservation trial in 1981. However there was a big difference as my group failed where they succeeded. The seeds of my failure were sown when I decided to publicly confront the issue of informed consent.

We were facing a remarkable ethical dilemma at this time. It is no exaggeration to claim that if a woman with breast cancer entered King's College Hospital and turned left into Lister ward on the first floor she would fall into the hands of surgeons who always did radical mastectomies with the best will in the world. If the said woman happened to turn right into Pantia Ralli ward she had as good a chance of falling into the hands of a surgical firm who with equal good will, believed beyond a shadow of doubt that breast conserving surgery was the treatment of choice. Neither group of surgeons were judged unethical because they truly believed they knew what was best.

However if this same woman were referred by her GP to see me then I would have expressed my uncertainty and at the time was publicly talking about launching a trial where the two same treatments were allocated at random in order to learn, for the benefit of future generations, the truth of the matter. This was judged unethical and in a debate on television with the editor of the Bulletin of Medical Ethics, I was compared to the "Beast of Belsen", Dr. Joseph Mengele, for daring to think about it. All this painfully demonstrated to me the double standards that existed at the time. If you treated all your patients the wrong way it was ethical but if you treated only half your patients the wrong way it was unethical! The trouble being that without the trial we would never learn what was right and what was wrong.

In the end I judged it beyond my expertise to progress alone so I appointed a very famous professor of radiotherapy to chair the steering committee and also recruited for the first time a lay ethicist to advise the steering committee. After much discussion under her leadership we published a long paper in the BMJ concerning the ethics of such a trial and concluded that as the outcomes were so dramatically different, then patient preferences however irrational or ill informed had to take precedence over the needs of society. For those reasons when we launched the trial much time was spent explaining the issues by word of mouth and written information leaflets, and only if the women appeared indifferent to the choice of treatment and provided written consent were we allowed to enter them into the trial. Well as you can guess very few women were indifferent and when we closed the trial after three years having only recruited 110 patients one of the medical journals described the event as "the trial that everyone needed but no one wanted". However in addition to what we had learnt about the ethics of consent and the double standards of routine clinical practice, something else of lasting value was garnered from the embers of failure. Very wisely, Lesley Fallowfield had set up a parallel study amongst the women in the trial in order to investigate the psychosocial consequences of the two extremes of treatment for breast cancer that had been allocated without bias. To do so meant developing a new set of psychometric instruments and capturing the women both before and at intervals after surgery. This way we learnt that about a third of the women irrespective of the treatment suffered from anxiety, depression and sexual dysfunction. It was of course hoped that preserving the breast might have improved psychological outcomes but what was learnt instead was that the existential threat to the woman trumped all other considerations and it was to take another 10 years before women accepted the safety of breast conserving surgery and could then start to benefit from the cosmetic advantage of retaining her breast. This pioneering work by Lesley and her colleagues set the scene for what today is commonplace, in that no major RCTs are likely to be funded unless a module is added to study the subjective outcomes of treatment and their impact on the patient's QOL.

There was however another ugly fallout from this study that nearly led to my suspension and haunts me to this day.

ET was a small middle-aged woman of unremarkable appearance but with the spark of intelligence in her eyes. She was referred to me by a local GP because she had recently become aware of a lump in her left breast. After a careful examination I broke the news to her that I suspected cancer. Following further tests I was convinced that the tumour was too large for her to be considered as a candidate for breast conserving surgery so when I next saw her I had to explain the need for a mastectomy and exploration of the glands in her armpit. On each occasion these consultations were witnessed by a few of my students who sat in on the clinics. She seemed to enjoy the fact that she was of value as a teaching aid and if I remember correctly I think she even volunteered for a demonstration at one of our weekly clinico-pathological teaching sessions. Along the way I genuinely felt that we had built a rapport and that she had come to trust me. The operation went well and she was discharged after only three days, but following a chance encounter with a fellow patient whilst waiting to see me at her next out patient appointment the roof fell in on me. She had learnt that the other patient had enjoyed the services of my counsellor and specialist nurse Sylvia Denton, something that she had been denied. Furthermore she had also learnt that she was acting as a "control" in a clinical trial to discover the psychological advantage of counselling sessions by a nurse. As a result of this she submitted her first formal complaint against me to the hospital authorities. What she didn't seem to appreciate was that I only had funds to support Sylvia part time and was taking advantage of the "natural experiment" of measuring the psychosocial outcomes of patients who were admitted on the days when Sylvia was in attendance with those who were admitted on the days when she was absent. Furthermore neither ET nor the hospital management seemed to understand that under my care patients had a fifty-fifty chance of some kind of psychological support whereas in the rest of London's hospitals there was zero chance. The fact that I was observing her as a subject in a study without her consent was an anathema. She then learnt about the CRC breast conservation trial that was still recruiting at King's and assumed that she had been randomized to a mastectomy in another trial without informed consent and would not accept my reassurances that the size of her tumour made her ineligible for the study. Nothing would satisfy her now except my suspension from the NHS. The next thing I knew was that she had gathered the support of a journalist who published a full-page article in the Sunday Observer entitled, "How secret trials abuse patients at a London teaching hospital". When interviewed about this a further report appeared with a picture of me looking like a stubborn version of Mussolini, with the caption, "Baum-no regrets".

After internal investigations the hospital agreed that I had no case to answer but that didn't satisfy her in the least, so her complaint went to a higher authority. A further full investigation with an independent committee set up by the regional health authority took place and once again I was exonerated; but that only served to inflame the matter further. She was able to persuade her local MP that there was a conspiracy afoot and he persuaded 40 MPs to place an early day motion in the House of Commons to debate the scandal. All of this ran on for about twelve months before she ran out of higher authorities to consider her case. In the meantime my reputation was tarnished and I became addicted to sleeping tablets.

With all such things there has to be two versions of the narrative I've described, but sadly the other version cannot be told as ET died of her breast cancer about 5 years after diagnosis. Yet I report the events as I remember them from 25 years ago, not so much as to portray myself as some kind of martyr to a cause but to illustrate by this vignette the ignorance and hostility with which the conduct of clinical trials was greeted in the early 1980s.

Chapter 11

1984 My Darkest Days!

---

*"It was the worst experience of my life. I was in a state that
bears no resemblance to anything I had experienced before.
I was not just feeling very low, depressed in the commonly
used sense of the word. I was seriously ill. I was totally self-
involved negative and thought about suicide all the time. I
could not think properly, let alone work, and wanted to remain
curled up in bed all day."*
Malignant Sadness, The Anatomy of Depression.
Lewis Wolpert, 1999
Faber & Faber

The dreadful quotation above comes from the opening paragraph
of a remarkable book by my friend and colleague Professor Lewis
Wolpert, Professor of Biology as Applied to Medicine at University
College London. He gifted me a copy as a token of thanks following
a dinner party at my house after we had been comparing notes on our
experiences of malignant sadness.

His description of what it felt like at the nadir of an episode of
acute depression is identical to my own experience, but how I reached
that point is worthy of a chapter in its own right as a warning to
others. How I recovered is a tribute to my wife and my doctors and
an illustration of personal growth out of adversity that might provide
hope for others afflicted with the illness.

A brief reiteration is required of the toxic environment that I had
built up for myself that provided a perfect culture medium for the

virus of depression to infect and progress unchecked. First of all my workload was indescribable and in retrospect an abuse of my human rights. In theory as a clinical professor I was supposed to apportion my time half and half between the NHS and the university. In practice like everyone else working for the NHS my good will was exploited and I carried the same burden as all my NHS colleagues. Furthermore out of sheer vanity I was determined to show that I was as good as any of them and not the stereotype professor of surgery "who couldn't cut himself out of a paper bag". That workload accounted for about 35 hours a week. A lot of my work concerned cancer and I never found it easy to break bad news. In addition I was on call for emergencies one night a week and one weekend in five. Often I would have to work through the night dealing with twisted guts, bleeding ulcers, perforated appendices, fractured skulls and the results of low intensity urban warfare on Coldharbour Lane, the road that leads directly from the back of my unit to the heart of Brixton, and affectionately referred to as "the front line". Next I was responsible for organizing the teaching of the undergraduates and taking my share of the lectures, teaching ward rounds and seminars. That accounted for about 15 hours a week. At that time I was also chairman of the board of examiners in surgery for the University of London's conjoint exam so that leading up to that summer of discontent I was in the examination halls for three days each week for nearly five weeks. Of course I had a large department to run and I had to compete for grants, as I was responsible for the welfare and career development of about 30 people. Reports had to written and papers had to be published in order to maintain or raise the profile of my academic unit. In the end I was working 11 hours a day on average including a full Saturday morning from 8.30 to 1.00pm. I took off Saturday afternoon and evening but worked at my papers all day Sunday. All this might have been just about supportable if I had no other worries and could look forward to a summer holiday. But we were penniless. By this time my two daughters were at private school as well so with three sets of school fees and a huge mortgage there was nothing left even for groceries and shoes, never mind a holiday. Judy went back to work and I even moonlighted as a GP in a practice in Camberwell Green. The summer of 1984 was hot but we couldn't afford to go away so I took a week off to carry out essential repairs and redecoration of the house. I had to relay a floor in the kitchen as the clock ticked away and my return to work unrested was all the worse for me having neglected it for a week of hard labour at home.

The week that followed is imprinted in my memory with the clarity of a high definition video film. Whilst I had been on "holiday" I was literally fattening up an emaciated woman for a major operation. This delightful lady of 65 years had been unable to swallow for about a month and had lost a lot of weight. The clinical and radiological diagnosis was simple: she had a cancer of the lower third of the oesophagus. Because of her state of malnutrition I started her on intravenous feeding with the idea of operating on her the day after I returned to work. My guilty secret was that I needed her as much as she needed me. My self-esteem was at an all time low but the chance of a relatively easy oesophagectomy, in a skinny but otherwise healthy woman, gave me the chance of a surgical "triumph" that might have gone some way to restoring my self image. I had even booked one of the scarce beds in the intensive care unit (ICU) without which the anaesthetist would not have allowed me to proceed. The night before the operation I had a blazing row over the phone with one of the cardio-thoracic surgeons who demanded that I gave up my ICU bed in favour of one of his more deserving patients. I wouldn't budge on this and went to bed seething and could only get off to sleep with a double dose of nitrazepam. The following morning, feeling dreadful, I accompanied my patient into the anaesthetic room holding her hand and offering reassurance. Just before I was to start, with the patient asleep and draped in green linen, there was an emergency call from ICU asking me to stay my hand as a young child with severe head injuries following a road traffic accident had just been admitted to "my bed".

I tore off my gloves and stormed out of theatre to check out on things in ICU with the forlorn hope that I might have been able to transfer one of these high dependency patients back to their own bed on the ward. It was hopeless as all of the ICU patients were on respirators. As I strode back to theatre I surprised and embarrassed myself by bursting into tears. I was then faced with the dilemma of what to do with my anaesthetised patient. I wasn't allowed to proceed with the planned procedure, so as a compromise I intubated the oesophageal stricture to provide her with a temporary passage for liquids to pass through. Of course it was me who had to break the news after she woke up and her family were less than pleased. Sadly I never had a second chance to operate and she went downhill thereafter.

The following day I had something to look forward to. I was scheduled to talk at the Oxford union and as the meeting would finish late I was going to stay with my brother David and sister-in-law Angela, in their North Oxford house. David was reader in Paediatrics at Oxford University at that time. After my talk I met up with my brother and enjoyed our first quality time together for ages, over a couple of pints of best bitter at the union bar. I went back to his place feeling warm and relaxed, hoping that I might sleep naturally that night having forgotten my pills. As the alcoholic haze wore off I was once again tormented by demons all night and never slept a wink. I got an early train back to London just in time to chair a difficult meeting at the Cancer Research Campaign HQ in Carlton House Terrace. I could barely concentrate and Richard Peto seemed to be droning on and on forever, as my head spun whilst he tried to explain esoteric statistical formulae. In the end I had to feign ill health and left the meeting early. Of course I was in fact seriously ill at the time without realizing it. The next morning I boarded the first train to Glasgow where I was scheduled to give a talk at a big meeting organized by the Royal College of Nurses. Shortly before the train was due to depart I was overcome by a sense of impending death. In a panic and to the dismay of my colleagues travelling with me, I leapt out of the train and grabbed a taxi to take me home, convinced that I was having a stroke. Poor Judy was terrified when I appeared suddenly looking wild eyed and dishevelled and she immediately sent for our GP as I strode up and down grabbing my hair and holding my chest. Of course you would have guessed by now that this was a panic attack but I was convinced that I was about to die.

Because of my past medical history my GP rapidly made the diagnosis of anxiety/depressive illness and my old friend and colleague Dr. Steven Greer, a psychiatrist at King's, made the first of a number of domiciliary visits. I was dosed up to the eyeballs with the antidepressant amitriptyline. This had the effect of sedating me so much that I slept for about 18 hours a day for the next week. The side effects of the drug were almost as bad as the disease. I wandered round like a zombie for the 6 weeks I was on maximum dose and I had a disgusting metallic taste in my mouth all the time that wasn't relieved by sucking peppermints. I woke up after a few days and was hit with the full realization of my condition and wept inconsolably. The miserable picture painted by Lewis Wolpert in the quotation that opens this chapter described my condition but I need to embellish it a little. I felt utterly worthless, like some kind of dog turd, and also felt that I was a pointless burden on my whole family. Every event and every kind and reassuring word was reinterpreted to support my delusion. The fact that so many friends and members of my family came to reassure me of my worth convinced me that I was a confidence trickster as well as a waste of space. People who have not experienced clinical depression can't begin to understand what it means. To use the vernacular it is not a feeling of being "pissed off", it is a feeling of utter helplessness, hopelessness and uselessness. Anyway after 6 weeks of drugs and behavioural therapy topped up by loving-kindness from my wife, kids and sibs, I started making a slow recovery. Once I was out of bed I started painting as art therapy. My early works were as dark and depressing as my mood. I destroyed them all later, but now I would like to illustrate the kind of thing I'm describing with a painting by a professional artist, Michel Petronie, who illustrated his cancer journey from the diagnosis of non-Hodgkin's lymphoma until shortly before his death after a second bone marrow transplant, with a remarkable series of paintings. (Figure 39) The one shown here is titled "can't see the wood for the trees" and the iconography is self-evident. Michel gave me this painting as a thank you after I helped stage a show of his work. Long before he had started on this work I had completed an identical composition although it lacked the vibrant colours of his painting. The first sign of my recovery was a painting of sunflowers in brilliant gold and yellows that is also shown here. (Figure 40)

Before I was allowed back to work the Dean, Mr. Len Cotton, a rather large and frightening vascular surgeon, insisted I took some additional paid leave, which was a true act of kindness.

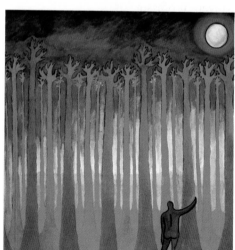

Fig. 39 "Can't see the wood for the trees", Michel Petronie

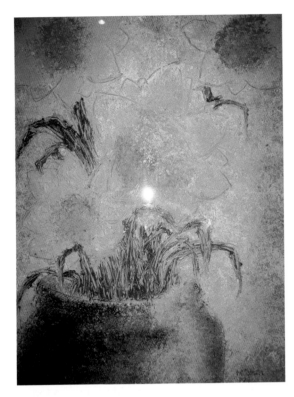

Fig. 40 Sunflowers, my own work, 1984

Shortly before I took ill I had been hosting a visiting professor in my department on sabbatical from Norway. This was Roar Nissen-Meyer, professor of radiation oncology at the University of Oslo. He was a lovely man and an unsung hero of breast cancer research. I learnt later that he was also an unsung hero of the Norwegian resistance to the Nazis. Shortly before the invasion Roar was sent to do his military service as a doctor in the north east of the country. During the occupation he acted for the resistance and radioed London with news about German troop movements at a time of the real threat of an invasion of the UK across the North Sea. Some Norwegian collaborator denounced him but he had about two hours notice of his intended arrest. Together with his wife Gerde and baby son in a sledge strapped to his waist, he escaped by skiing across the mountains into Sweden, making the border just ahead of the German pursuit. He and his family were flown to Scotland where he trained as an agent and was parachuted back into Norway to continue spying on the German army. He escaped with his life and later on was decorated for bravery by the King of Norway. I think I'm the only one to have been shown his medals outside his family. As far as his heroism in breast cancer research he could claim perhaps three firsts. He was the first to set up multicentre collaboration in clinical trials by establishing the Nordic oncology network. He was the first to show the benefit of oophorectomy in the adjuvant treatment of breast cancer and he was one of the first to trial adjuvant chemotherapy. Roar was a slim neat man, very fit from all that cross-country skiing and very modest. Judy and I became firm friends of Roar and Gerde. When they learnt of my plight they insisted that we came for a fortnight of complete rest in their summer-house (hüt) on an island in the Oslo fiord. This sounded idyllic and timely.

Judy packed for all weathers as well as the odd cocktail dress and matching heels. I packed for a holiday on a remote island. I was the clever one. The Nissen-Meyers met us at the airport and drove to where they had moored their boat. We sailed across the fiord and landed at a rocky promontory near to their hut. It was the funniest of sights to witness Roar and myself carrying four suitcases across the rocks to this isolated hut on an otherwise uninhabited island. Roar and Gerde arranged to stay the night with us in order to settle us in. Gerde explained that the nearest co-operative shop was on the mainland about half an hour across the fiord in a westerly direction but we needn't worry, as their island was self-sufficient. For example there was the vegetable garden just by the side of the water and there was a cod in the fridge that would be good for two days until Michael caught some more fish.

Judy, my Jewish princess, blanched at the thought of having to gut a freshly caught cod. I blanched as I recalled that I had never knowingly caught a fish in my life.

I mentioned this to Roar and he said I would be fine and demonstrated how to catch fish by laying out a net from the easterly edge of the island to a rock 100 meters out. The net was loaded on a rowing boat and dropped over the side until I reached the rock where it could be tied to a post driven into the granite.

After a jolly evening eating cod and fresh vegetables washed down with beer and schnapps our host and hostess left us to our own devices. The next day I relaxed and sketched in the balmy sunshine, whilst Judy cooked cod and fresh vegetables. About noon I heard a scream from a wooden outhouse. One thing the Nissen-Meyers had forgotten to mention was that the indoor flushing toilet was in fact out of doors and did not flush. Who needs to flush when you have a deep dark hole in the ground? Another thing I've forgotten to tell you about Judy is that she suffers from arachnophobia. Arachnoids favour deep dark holes in the ground and yes you've guessed the rest. Having beaten off the 8-legged monster and sprayed the hole with a can with a label that read something like "Araachïnïdmörtengësheften", she was appeased but warned me not to expect to make that journey at night. That evening I took the little boat (Figure 41) and laid the net, more in hope than expectation, and returned to the hut for an early night as there was nothing else to do, and the only Norwegian TV service that we could pick up ran only from 6.00 p.m. to 10.00 p.m. Judy sat up all night too terrified to sleep, not because of the fear of spiders, but because of the fear of being 30 miles away from the nearest neighbours, and with a husband who couldn't navigate the sailing dinghy left for our personal use.

The next morning I took the rowboat out to the rock with my wife, arms akimbo, looking on sceptically, and started hauling in the net. To my delight I saw that I had caught two beautiful large cod, to my surprise on hauling in another metre of net I saw a further three magnificent cod, and to my growing horror I realized that I had caught a whole shoal of north sea cod.

As I lugged the damp net and the many many kilos of fish into the boat it started to sink under the weight. We only just made it back to the island as the North Sea slurped over the gunnels into the hull of the boat. It took the two of us to unburden the boat and bale it out. I spent the whole day disengaging fish from the net with their baleful fish eyes staring at me with hatred. My hands were cut and bleeding at the end of this exhausting exercise and most of the

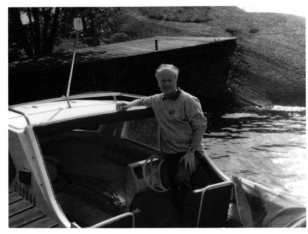

Fig. 41 Me catching cod in Norway

133

catch was returned to where it belonged. We kept two large cod in the fridge and Judy cooked another delicious meal of freshly caught fish and fresh garden vegetables. After a couple more days we at last recognized something previously unknown about our characters. We are not country folk, we are not of fishermen stock, we are not at home in the wilderness and we like company, lots of it. In the end, the benefits of escaping the solitude and the cabin madness were outweighed by the hazard of sailing a little boat to the mainland in search of a hotel with people, noise, indoor flushing toilets and above all a change from cod du jour plus boiled carrots. We packed one case and sailed away from the island without another boat in sight and with my only knowledge of handling a sailing boat from what I remembered of Arthur Ransome's "Swallows and Amazons" that I had read as a boy. Fortunately no sudden squalls blew up and entirely by luck we drifted into a jetty on the western edge of the fiord where we checked into a perfectly decent hotel. We enjoyed the rest of our stay and sneaked back the way we came, just in time to warmly greet the Nissen-Meyers as they arrived to pick us up and return us to the airport. Not a word of our adventures would they ever hear and we remained good friends for a decade or so.

On returning home I suddenly recognized that I was looking forward to returning to my work and the break had served me well. My mental health was also improved by the fact that my friendly Nat West bank manager had agreed to a loan that would consolidate all my debts and pay for the school fees in advance. He told me that he had every confidence in me, and my future earning capacity. I'm happy to say that I honoured the trust he placed in me.

They say that hard work never killed anybody; that's not true. It nearly killed me, and certainly contributed to the premature death of my brother David.

I learnt some other important lessons from this episode. A work/life balance is important for everyone and the Jewish laws concerning the Sabbath were the first to recognize this truism. I learnt that you can't please all the people all the time and you must say no when others wish to burden you with work beyond your capacity. I learnt that the NHS cares little for the welfare of its staff and makes no provision for caring for the carers. Finally I learnt what depression means and the fact that up to 30% of my patients had to put up with it was just unacceptable. Although I can't genuinely empathize with a woman about to lose her breast I sure as hell can empathize with her when I spot the first symptoms of impending malignant sadness.

Chapter 12

The Royal Marsden
Hospital 1989–2000

After my return to work at King's I remained on amytriptaline for another 6 months still feeling vulnerable but mercifully free of panic attacks. Within a few days after Dr. Greer said I could stop the treatment I felt my old self and could start tasting my food again. To avoid making the mistakes of the past and in order to reduce my burden of work I gradually gave up general surgery in order to concentrate on breast cancer. As my reputation in this subject grew I was starting to have private patients referred from amongst the great and the good. Of course the university rules meant that I couldn't pocket the money, which had to go to support my department, but I could at least keep the gifts and I did meet some exotic creatures. One gift from a grateful sheik was a gold Rolex with the sheik's head engraved upon its face. The family judged it to be too vulgar to wear so I pawned it in exchange for a summer holiday for the family. Not long after that I got another Rolex, much more tasteful than the last, from another grateful monarch of a Gulf state. At that time most of my senior colleagues sported what we had come to describe as "Gulf watches". My son wears that one to this day as it was replaced by the Rolex I was awarded as part of the St Gallen prize for a lifetime achievement in breast cancer research in 2007.

However the most exotic experience of that kind followed the referral of the senior wife of the Sultan of an Islamic state. Whilst I operated on her breast two of the Sultan's armed guards were stationed at the door to the theatre. I seem to recall that they bore curved scimitars but that just might have been a flight of my imagination.

She made an excellent recovery and before her departure the finance minister of the Sultanate came to pay me for my trouble. He carried a large Gladstone bag and was also escorted by armed guards. When he asked me my fee I had no idea what the going rate was so mentioned the first large sum that came into my head; "Ermmm-would £500 be OK?" The minister opened his bag, split one of about 20 bundles of notes in two and gave me my £500 from what looked like a kitty of £20,000. That helped pay for new carpets in my department whilst those at home grew more threadbare.

About 12 months later I was invited to one of the Sultan's palaces in that far away land to check up on HRH the senior Sultana. As all my expenses were being paid and I was being treated as a VIP, I took the missus along for the ride. It was red carpets and chauffeur-driven Mercedes all round with a glamorous dinner hosted by the minister of health on the evening of our arrival. The following day we were shown into the presence of HRH the Sultan and whilst I went upstairs to visit my patient the Sultan entertained Mrs. Baum. This "entertainment" consisted of him showing Judy photographs of himself from childhood all the way through to his magnificence in the full regalia of his coronation, whilst placing his hand on her knee. *Afterwards he offered me 6 camels in exchange for Judy if she would enter his harem. I paused just a beat too long, to Judy's barely controlled rage***. Just to show that he took this in good humour he presented me with a silver dish engraved with his likeness. As I was about to leave the self same minister of finance stopped me to ask about my fee. Having learnt from my mistake of the past I explained that I wanted nothing for myself but that £20,000 for my breast cancer research wouldn't go amiss. He replied with a sigh to the effect that under any other circumstances he would have said yes but the state's exchequers were empty, as the huge mosque the Sultan had just endowed had run over the estimates by a large amount. The last minute decision to cover the dome in gold leaf was a big mistake.

I left empty handed but Judy and I could barely stop giggling as we made our dignified exit.

On a more serious note the two most important themes of my last few years at King's, (which would impact on the rest of my career), should be mentioned in passing. Both of these themes justify chapters

---

**That bit is a "factoid", in other words not actually true but to give a colour and flavour to the episode.

of their own, as their relevance and ongoing development continue to this day.

The first of these was my run-in with HRH the Prince of Wales over the subject of alternative medicine in 1985 (see chapter 17) and the second concerns the establishment of the first breast cancer screening unit in the south east of England that fell to my responsibility in 1987 (see chapter 16).

In 1989 I was invited to the chair of surgery at the Royal Marsden Hospital (RMH) and the Institute of Cancer Research (ICR). This was an offer I could hardly refuse.

Having been invited I could to a modest extent determine my own terms and conditions, which included the right to a modest private practice of my own. The RMH/ICR was considered a centre of excellence and one of the most prestigious specialist cancer units in Europe. I could now truly focus on my specialist subject and enjoy an infrastructure that supported research. Finally by being at a post-graduate institution I would be released from my burden of teaching medical students and the additional burden of organizing the curriculum and the examinations.

The RMH and ICR are housed on two sites. The first on Fulham Road, Chelsea, and the second at Sutton, a one and a half hour drive through the worst of south west London's traffic. This crazy arrangement had a historical precedent that I can't recall. My department and clinical facilities were at the Chelsea campus conveniently close to the rather decadent Chelsea Arts Club that was quick to welcome me as one of the few non-professional artist members. (Their "tarts and vicars" parties were great fun but that's not really relevant to this narrative.) I was once again successful in raising a large grant from a charitable foundation that allowed me to build a nice suite of offices and a set of laboratories. I had a wonderful set of colleagues who became lifelong friends and because of our international reputation we were able to attract the best of the best post-graduate students from all over the world. The next five years were amongst the happiest and fulfilling years of my life until once again NHS reorganization spoilt it all. I'll return to that at the end of the chapter. As one of the new boys I was entitled to ask for new toys, so I set up the latest video technology for sharing pathology and X ray pictures in a refurbished seminar room in order to house a weekly multidisciplinary clinico-pathology conference. I will expand on this in the chapter "The school of Athens", but suffice to say that this forum for intellectual debate on the diagnosis and treatment of cancers, containing some of the best brains in the world, attracted huge audiences and were the highlight of my working week.

Amongst my closest friends and colleagues were Professor Mitch Dowsett, head of endocrinology, Professor Iain Smith, a professor of medicine, and Professor Trevor Powles, a brilliant medical oncologist. We used to argue passionately amongst ourselves and then take off for a friendly pint of beer at the local pub, "The Princess of Wales". If I got home late for dinner and the worse for wear I would always blame it on the bad company I had fallen in with. It was worse when professor Tony Howell from Manchester was in town or if we had professor John Forbes visiting from the land of Oz, but each one added to the intellectual buzz and creativity of the place. Talking of the Princess of Wales, the real one, aka Lady Diana, she was one of our Patrons. Later on when I became clinical director it was my privilege to conduct her round the wards. Her visits were kept a secret but my wife always suspected something when I returned home with a fresh haircut and a silly smile on my face. She even graced the opening ceremony of my new laboratories and looked down one of my microscopes at one of my cell cultures. It was love at first sight, not the princess and the cell culture, but me and the princess. My love might have been reciprocated but I think she found me a little too short and too fat for her taste. There was one remarkable occasion when I had to operate on an old lady who returned to her bed on my ward half an hour before a royal visit. As the princess approached the bed and I started to explain what the old woman had just gone through, HRH stretched forward to hold the old dear's gnarled hand at which the old dear woke with a start and without missing a beat smiled from ear to ear and said, "'Allo Lady Di watchyer adoin 'ere then?" There is no doubt that the princess loved these visits and they did wonders for the morale of staff and patients alike.

Without doubt the most important component of my work over the 5 years I spent at the RMH/ICR was the development and launching of the ATAC trial.

To understand the significance of this I will have to back off a bit and describe some simple facts about endocrinology.

My laboratories were next door to those of Professor Mitch Dowsett, world leader in the field of hormones and breast cancer. He was one of the pioneers in the understanding of the mechanisms of action of tamoxifen. The endocrine system consists of all the glands that produce hormones such as the thyroid that produces thyroxine, the pituitary that produces growth hormone and the ovaries that produce oestrogen in premenopausal women. In postmenopausal women oestrogens can be detected in the circulation but at levels about ten times lower than in younger women. The origin of oestrogens in older women was a mystery until about 20 years ago. In the end it was discovered that the adrenal glands that sit on top of the kidneys and are responsible for producing cortisone also produce low levels of the male hormone testosterone in low concentrations. This male hormone is then metabolized in the fatty tissue of women via an enzyme known as *aromatase,* to produce oestrogen. This is essential to maintain skeletal health in postmenopausal women. All target tissues that respond to hormones have a protein in their cells that bind the hormone and present the complex to the DNA within the nucleus. These binding proteins are called receptors and for the purpose of this story we should concentrate on the oestrogen receptor (ER) and the progesterone receptor (PgR) that are both involved in the proliferation and function of normal breast epithelial cells.

About 75% of breast cancer cells retain this mechanism and are referred to as hormone responsive. (Figure 42) Hormone responsive breast cancers stop proliferating and start to die if deprived of oestrogen.

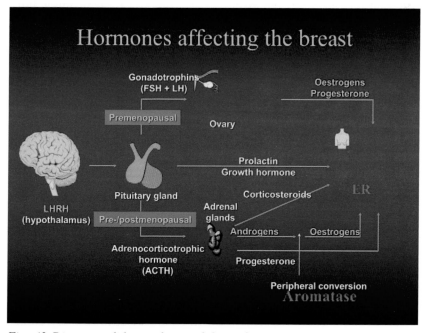

Fig. 42 Diagram of the workings of the endocrine system

Tamoxifen was developed as an anti-oestrogen but had a paradoxical effect of stimulating the ovaries. Mitch Dowsett's work went someway to explain this in showing that like Janus, the two faced God of ancient Greece, tamoxifen had both agonist as well as antagonist effects. As far as the breast cancer cells were concerned the drug acted as an antioestrogen but as far as the endometrial cells in the uterus and the osteoblasts in the skeleton the drug was seen as an agonist (stimulant). This then accounted for two side effects of tamoxifen, one favourable and the other unfavourable, in postmenopausal women. The favourable side effect was the protection of the skeleton from osteoporosis and the unfavourable was the stimulus of the endometrium leading to postmenopausal bleeding and rarely endometrial cancer.

In the meantime the pharmaceutical industry had developed pure aromatase inhibitors (AIs) that in theory could shut down oestrogen production completely in the older woman. These drugs were investigated in the lab by Mitch and in the clinic by Trevor Powles.

As our labs were close to each other we shared a coffee room and our conversations strayed to consider the possibility of an AI being superior to tamoxifen as adjuvant therapy for early breast cancer. Early experience with the AIs showed that they were extremely well tolerated and active in the advanced disease. On a train coming back from (I think) Edinburgh after a meeting of the BBG, a group of us that included Joan Houghton, Jeff Tobias, Tony Howell, Mitch and myself, designed the ideal trial on the back of a coffee stained envelope. Jeff kept the envelope and here it is reproduced. (Figure 43)

We hawked this idea around the pharmaceutical companies producing the AIs and Astra Zeneca (AZ) accepted our ideas with the obvious proviso that we used their drug *anastrozole* (Arimidex). This involved a great leap of faith, as we had yet no idea if Arimidex was more effective in the advanced disease than tamoxifen. The trial involved randomizing postmenopausal women with operable breast cancer to Arimidex (A), Tamoxifen (T) Alone or Combined (AC), hence the acronym ATAC. One third of the women would get A one third T and one AT. AZ were to provide the drugs free and finance the infrastructure for the trial in the CRC clinical trials unit but an independent international steering committee would supervise the conduct of the trial and independent of that would be a data monitoring and safety committee (DMSC) who had the power to stop the study if there was any suggestion of statistically significant differences in serious adverse events or efficacy between any two of the three arms.

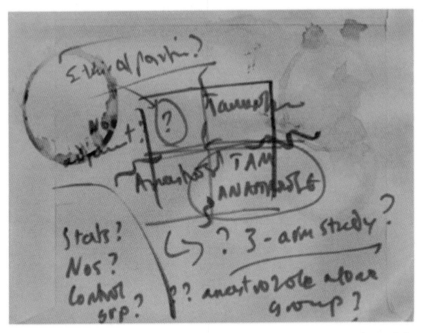

Fig. 43 the brown paper envelope on which is described the outline of the ATAC trial, which recruited over 9,000 patients and discovered something better than tamoxifen

This trial was hugely ambitious as we were challenging the "gold standard" of cancer treatment for this class of patient. Secondly we were looking for evidence not only of improved effectiveness in cancer outcomes but also improvements in toxicity and tolerability so that in the end we might draw up a balance sheet of benefits versus harms. To achieve this we had to overcome some awesome statistical hurdles, so at this point a short diversion is required.

If you toss a coin the odds of it coming down heads or tails are 50:50. If you throw a dice the odds of it coming up with any given number of spots is one in six. When you play contract bridge you know that in the fullness of time both you and your partner will average out 10 points per hand. When tossing a coin often enough you might come up with an impressive run of heads or tails, say 15 heads out of 25 tosses. Simple mathematics of probability theory will show that this is not significant and to draw a conclusion that the coin is bent or the tosser is bent is called a type 1 (alpha) error. If you throw a pair of dice 12 times and they come up double six

6 times you know the dice have been tampered with and that is a significant departure from the laws of probability.

If you and your partner consistently pick up balanced hands with less than 6 points for three months at a time then that's contract bridge as played in my house where the laws of probability seem suspended.

All of this applies to comparing cancer treatment when we try to discount differences in outcome if they could be accounted for by the play of chance, even if that chance is only one in twenty; described as $p<0.05$. The statistical tests used have the function of excluding the type 1 error. However there is another error due to the play of chance that is equally important i.e. missing a clinically significant result as a result of the sample size in the trial being too small. That is known as a type 2 (beta) error. Here the mathematics gets a bit complex but trust me when I state that there is a 20% chance of missing a 5% difference in breast cancer recurrence rates even with a trial of over a thousand patients. We describe this factor as the power of the trial. No one would wish to launch a very expensive and important trial with such an important chance of failure.

We therefore "powered up" the ATAC trial so that there was only a 10% chance of missing a clinically important result (i.e. 90% power) whilst also having the power to detect important differences in predetermined toxic side effects. Ultimately our chief of statistics, Professor Jack Cuzick, came up with the sobering news that we would need over 9,000 patients or in other words over 3,000 patients in each arm of the study. Strictly speaking the power in the trial isn't in the number of patients recruited but the number of patients you predict might experience an "event" over say the next five years. The first "event" of interest would be recurrence of breast cancer, but if the control group is already taking tamoxifen with a predicted 5-year recurrence free rate of about 75% we were setting ourselves a high bar to clear. To recruit 9,000 patients within a reasonable time period was a huge and expensive challenge.

Astra Zeneca were well aware that their competitors Novartis and Pfizer were hot on their heels so they plunged in with a major financial gamble and gave us the green light. With adequate funding we were able to rapidly recruit the staff to support the trial at home and abroad and once again I packed my bags to set off on the first of a number of global travels to recruit centres from all round the world for this massive task. It took all my powers of diplomacy to persuade new centres that they were equal stakeholders and to an extent this was achieved by a publication policy that would recognize everyone's contributions equally. The main publications were to be in the name of the ATAC trialist group with a very long appendix naming all centres and all contributors. In the end we recruited from 381 centres in 21 countries making it the largest collaborative effort in clinical cancer research on record.

The travel involved in order to hold the group together was exhausting and British Airways eventually rewarded me with a gold executive card. In the name of fair play our international steering committee meeting that gathered three times a year met once in London and the other two times in either Europe or North America. Professor Aman Buzdar from the M D Anderson Cancer Centre Houston Texas was our man in America and was responsible for a huge effort in recruiting over 2,000 patients; whilst my old mate Professor John Forbes in Newcastle NSW was our man at the ANZ breast group in Australia, that "boxed well above their weight". I loved my visits to the wonderful world of Oz but hated the journey getting there. In the end I was familiar with Sydney, Melbourne, Perth, Brisbane, Darwin and Cairns. There were very few punters from the red-hot centre of that red continent.

We reached our target in about three years and I was able to report our preliminary results at the premier breast cancer event, the San Antonio Breast Cancer Symposium, in 2001. Standing up in front of an expectant audience of about 10,000 of my peers, I thought a little theatre might be in order as I only had 10 minutes to put the message across. 5 minutes was used up describing the rationale, methodology and statistics of the study. The first result slide (Figure 44) showed the "life table" curves for recurrence-free survival i.e. percent of patients in each cohort alive and free of cancer recurrence. As a tease I showed the curve for tamoxifen and then after a pause of a second or two I unfolded the result for anatrozole that needless to say was significantly superior. After I sat down the audience went mad and I savoured the moment that is maybe experienced once in a lifetime by only a minority of scientists. Funnily enough I didn't feel the least bit smug or complacent. In fact I felt a sense of caution whilst at the same time remembering the "wounds of battle" I'd suffered on the road to this point.

The result I described was only the headline but it did translate into an absolute improvement of a modest 2.5% chance of a woman being recurrence-free at 5 years after surgery.

A few more details are needed here to make sense out of a massive set of data. First of all, the combined arm A+T was no better

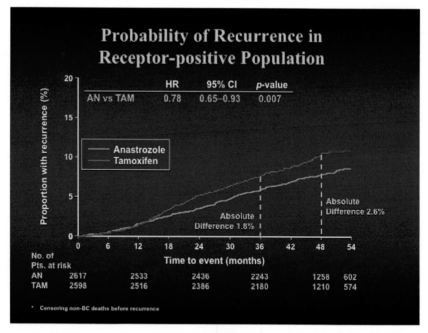

Fig. 44 The first results from the ATAC trial

than T alone and was therefore abandoned. Although this result was counter-intuitive Mitch Dowsett eventually was able to explain it in his laboratory models. It appeared that in an oestrogen-deprived environment as achieved by an aromatase inhibitor in a postmenopausal woman, the cancer cells use tamoxifen as an agonist instead of an antagonist. This again is an example of the importance of the scientific method on "setting limits to our ignorance". Next, this time expected, the benefits of A were confined to the ER+ group of patients. The toxicity profiles of the two drugs were strikingly different. Tamoxifen was associated with more gynaecological problems that lead to a four-fold excess of hysterectomies and in addition an increase in the risk of thrombosis. In contrast although anastrozole was better tolerated in the short term its use was associated with an increased risk of osteoporosis and fractures. In addition the patients described an increase in joint pain (polyarthralgia) and vaginal dryness. However to put all this into perspective only 7% of the patients on anastrozole had to stop taking the drug because of side effects and the group as a whole enjoyed a 92% chance of remaining recurrence-free at 5 years. Furthermore the most important side effect of the aromatase inhibitor can be dealt with by avoiding its use in women who are osteoporotic at the time of diagnosis and in monitoring the bone density (BMD) annually in the remainder. If the BMD falls there are a number of agents that can be used (bisphosphanates) to reverse this trend. After all we don't withhold chemotherapy for fear of a drop in white cell count, we anticipate the event and correct it should it occur.

With further maturation of the data the American Society of Clinical Oncology changed its guidelines and Astra Zeneca started enjoying a return on its investment. Our latest results at 10 year's follow up with all patients having completed their 5 year treatment shows the curves in recurrence-free survival continuing to diverge with about a 5% absolute difference (approximately 25% relative risk reduction) favouring Arimidex. Other trials of other AIs (Novartis' letrozole and Pfizer's exemestane) have shown similar outcomes and there now remains a turf war concerning whether any one of the three available AI's is superior to the other. Personally I think it unlikely. The other unresolved issue is whether two years of tamoxifen followed by three years of an AI is superior to 5 years of an AI, but this is all fine-tuning that follows any scientific breakthrough. As of today the National Institute of Clinical Excellence in the UK (NICE) recommends that all postmenopausal women with ER+ breast cancers should receive an AI as part of their care.

Of course whilst all this excitement was going on I still had a daytime job and that was starting once more to prove problematical. In 1999, once again the hospital services in London were seen as ripe for another re-disorganization, the 17th I personally experienced. This time Professor Tomlinson, a professor of pathology from Newcastle-upon-Tyne, was put in charge. No wonder pathologists are referred to as morbid anatomists! He looked at the map and noted far too many hospitals in west central London so he placed a red cross against the RMH. The Tomlinson report provoked a fierce response by simply failing to accept the notion of an internationally famous centre of excellence. No NHS hospital was permitted to be more equal than another. Under the chairmanship of Duke Hussey, director general of the BBC and chairman of our own board, I joined a gang of four to mount a campaign to save the RMH.

Over the next few months a bitter battle ensued. My friend and colleague Mr. Alan McKenna, a brilliant and kindly breast cancer surgeon, decided that now was the time to take an early retirement. Another one of my colleagues at the Sutton branch suffered a stroke and my friend and senior lecturer, Nigel Sacks, the one who had cared for my sister, decided to move to St George's as he feared for his financial future with a young family to support. In the light of the uncertainty about its future the hospital was unwilling to reappoint to these three vacancies and I was left being responsible for the work of four surgeons. Things eventually came to a head when I received a letter signed by the *deputy* complaints manager that read: " It has come to my notice that an increasing number of patients have been complaining of not meeting a consultant in person when attending the breast unit. How do you intend to address this problem?" I responded by suggesting that if we employed one less complaints manager and one more surgeon we might just get by, but sadly my irony was not appreciated. Then I experienced the first symptoms of a panic attack in 4 years. This time however there was a functioning health care system for the hospital employees. I took myself off right away to see the lovely Dr. Anne Fingret, head of occupational therapy. She was appalled at my story and started me on a programme of stress control without redress to drugs. I was just about coping with her support but she warned me that I couldn't go on with my current workload. I then wrote to our chief executive that unless another surgeon was appointed within six weeks I would have to resign. Of course one never threatens to resign unless you have a bolthole and as chance would have it I had just been made the offer of a personal chair at University College London. I waited for six weeks without even having an acknowledgment of my letter, and in spite of the entreaties from my friends and colleagues on the staff, I once again swapped chairs.

In 2002 I was awarded the William McGuire award at the annual San Antonio Breast Cancer symposium, the highest recognition for breast cancer research in the USA, for my work on adjuvant endocrine therapy. In subsequent years Trevor Powles and Mitch Dowsett were also honoured in this way. Three British citizens from the same institution winning a top American award must tell you something about centres of excellence, yet the Royal Marsden Hospital was in peril of closure by the NHS, a body that doesn't recognize excellence and is managed by bean counters trying to meet targets set by governments without consultation with those who actually know a thing or two about cancer.

Chapter 13

The School of Athens: UCL 2000–2005

During my years as professor at University College London I always looked forward to Tuesday morning as the highlight of my working week. I would arrive at the Middlesex hospital at 07.30 am to park my car, pop into the offices of the academic department of surgery in Riding House Street, to collect my notes and then start my extraordinary odyssey to the multidisciplinary meeting (MDM) at University College Hospital, followed by the breast cancer clinic at the Elizabeth Garret Anderson Hospital next to Euston station.

Riding House Street as its name suggests used to be occupied by the mews serving the needs of the gentry in the grand Georgian houses of Fitzrovia. The upper classes of 18thC London considered it fashionable to employ black servants. One of these, Olaudah Equiano (1745–1797) known as "The African", used to live in the building now occupied by the department of surgery. His autobiography describing the suffering and barbarity of the slave trade, published in 1789, helped pave the way for the abolitionists. A plaque describing these events is still to be seen over the door at number 72.

I would then walk east between the soot-stained walls of the back of the Middlesex Hospital and the even grimmer walls of the old workhouse that until recently served as the outpatient facility. A quick dogleg along Tottenham Street would bring me to the junction of one of London's busiest thoroughfares, Tottenham Court Road. At this corner lies a curious little square open to the main road, one of the last unreconstructed gaps left by the blitz of London in 1941. The square is backed by a wall marking the end of a row of once humble terrace houses now given over to boutiques. This wall is covered by a three storey badly painted and hideous mural illustrating the evils of war and the threat of a nuclear disaster. Costa Coffee serving the best cappuccino in the neighbourhood marks the northern limit of this little square. Every Tuesday morning at 07.45 am I would encounter "The School of Athens", as I called them, drinking not coffee, but Tennents strong lager. The one with the long scraggy beard and long grey locks I privately named Aristotle, the one with patched tartan trousers and much body piercing I named Plato, the one with the string vest (in all weathers) and ferocious tattoos I named Socrates and the filthy bag woman I christened Minerva the goddess of wisdom.

Whenever I approached them they were always enjoying an animated debate with much gesticulation that from a distance seemed to emulate the body language of scholarly disputation. God alone knows what profanities and idiocies were being proclaimed by their alcohol-sodden, foul smelling, early morning mouths and what passed for thinking in their addled brains, but from a distance they looked wise. This corner of London, as described in Peter Ackroyd's wonderful history of our remarkable city, has always been the home of the street people, sleeping rough, begging and drinking or drugging themselves to an early grave. My "School of Athens" looked to have an average age of 80 but were more likely to be in their early forties. Our A&E departments were full of them in the winter months with frost-bitten gangrenous toes, pneumonia or tuberculosis or with terminal haemorrhage from oesophageal varicose, a consequence of cirrhosis of the liver. Our medical students were privileged, if that's the right word, to study third world disease at the centre of one of the Western world's richest metropolises.

How could this be allowed?

Turning the corner onto Tottenham Court Road, I would encounter another rough sleeper and his dog on his patch conspicuously close to the cash point at my local bank. As he begged for enough to buy a cup of tea I would immediately be thrown into a whirlpool of contradictory impulses. At first the angel on my right shoulder would urge me to give him a pound, after all I wouldn't miss it and at least a hot drink on a cold day like today might stave off his death for another 24 hours. Then the angel on my left shoulder would shout, "Don't be stupid Michael, you know he won't spend it on a cuppa, it will only go towards his next fix and why does he have to beg in any case when the welfare state should be providing him unemployment and social security benefits". In the end the decision was made simply on the ease with which I could find a pound coin in my pocket that morning. If I paid up I felt a sucker and if I didn't pay up I felt like Scrooge. It was always a no win situation that would leave me unsettled until I crossed the road and turned north for a few blocks before turning east into University Street. Those last few blocks on Tottenham Court Road also left me musing about another set of unfortunates who plied their trade in this square mile. All the telephone boxes in this area have their walls plastered with calling cards of young women who are scantily dressed and adopting provocative poses so as to display their assets. Again I would be thrown into confusion. Why, if indeed these were genuine likenesses, did such gorgeous girls have to sell themselves? Surely there must be hundreds of young men willing to make honest women of them; and who were the sad old men that needed their services? Finally how dare they thrust their pneumatic bosoms in my face on a morning when I would no doubt be explaining to some other woman why she would have to lose one of her breasts? Eventually, after having run this gauntlet of emotions, I would arrive at the junction of University Street and Gower Street, opposite the Jeremy Bentham pub, named after the founder of our university. On entering the department of pathology peace would settle on me again as I looked forward to the amiable company of some truly wise and scholarly colleagues at the weekly MDM.

The pathology conference room was set up in a very structured manner. "On stage" front left the pathologists would command the microscopes and the projection equipment that would display their hugely magnified images on the screen. Stage right the radiologists would control the video cameras that could project magnified views of the mammograms onto the video screen.

Front left in the audience the most junior doctor of the team would present the case histories and record the details of our discussions for future audit using PowerPoint on a PC also projected on the screen. The consultant surgeons, radiotherapists and medical oncologists together with any visiting dignitaries occupied the front row of the stalls. The junior medical staff in each of these disciplines occupied second row of the stalls. Third row held the clinical nurse specialists and interested lab staff, whilst the back two rows by tradition were for the yawning, puking and mewling medical students, resenting this early hour. I acted as a cross between music hall master of ceremonies and agent provocateur. The mutual affection and respect of the consultants for each other was demonstrated by their locker room geniality, point scoring and friendly teasing. If foreign visitors were present this was exaggerated for effect. Yet in all honesty individual patients were discussed with the greatest of respect and confidentiality, in the greatest detail, with enormous scholarship, by a group of experts who were often to be seen delivering key note lectures at international meetings ranging from San Antonio, Texas, to ASCO in Chicago, EBCC Barcelona, via Milan and St. Gallen, Switzerland. This is something the NHS should be truly proud of, yet I'm sure our political masters were totally unaware that we were starting our working day an hour earlier than contracted, out of sheer professionalism.

It is hard to convey the enthusiasm surgeons display in the study of pathology (also known as morbid anatomy) in their chosen discipline. Certainly for me and I'm sure for others, there is an aesthetic as much as a scientific interest in the subject. To try and capture your interest I will start with the aesthetics of the subject by describing the exquisite microscopic anatomy and molecular biology of the normal breast before trying to explain the malignant transformation that literally turns this transcendental beauty into life-threatening ugliness.

First of all it is necessary to say something about *fractal* geometry as a jumping-off point for a description of normality. A *fractal* is a geometric shape that shares self-similar intricate structures on all scales of magnification.

As chance would have it last night I went to see Tom Stoppard's play, "Arcadia" for the second time. Towards of the end of the second act, set in 1809, we see a very precocious 13 year-old girl, Thomasina, talking to her tutor Septimus. Whilst discussing Newton's determinism she comes to an intuitive realization that there must be some kind of mathematical formula that when solved would define the shape of the branching leaf on the apple that concussed Newton.

> *"God's truth, Septimus, if there is an equation for a curve like a bell, there must be an equation for one like a blue bell, and if a bluebell why not a rose? Do we believe nature is written in numbers?"*

Her workbooks, discovered 200 years later by one of her direct descendants who just happens to be a brilliant Cambridge mathematician, demonstrate that she had hit upon the essential feature of non-linear mathematics or chaos theory. Sadly for Thomasina, there were no computers available to carry out the thousands of iterations of the algorithm that would reproduce not just a leaf but also a whole weeping willow on my desktop i-Mac. This type of mathematics can explain all the morphologies of the biological world, both its flora and its fauna. It is not by chance that the structure of a sprig of broccoli almost perfectly reflects the structure of the bronchial tree. (Figures 45, 46)

Whenever I eat broccoli I go into some kind of reverie about this and once when my wife fed me a mutant form of broccoli with elongated gaps between each branch I went so far as to write to the supermarket HQ asking if anyone there knew of the genetic differences between the two variants as it might provide a clue to the first step in malignant transformation. Needless to say I got no reply. On another occasion as a joke I got my friendly pathologist, Mary Falzon, to cut a section of the vegetable, stain it and mount it on a slide. She showed it at the annual Christmas quiz and we gave a prize of a bottle of wine for the best answer. I think "multifocal low grade veginoma" won the day. Broccoli, as well as resembling the bronchial tree, is an almost perfect representation of the mammary ducts and glands at the time of lactation.

The main difference of course is that the branches of the mammary gland are tubular. Imagine a tree-like tubular structure and then imagine taking transverse or random oblique cut sections and magnify them up. If the structure is perfectly symmetrical and the cuts are

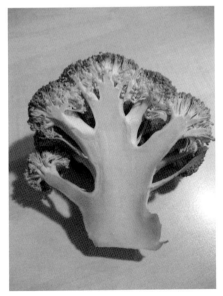

Fig. 45 Fractal geometry of broccoli

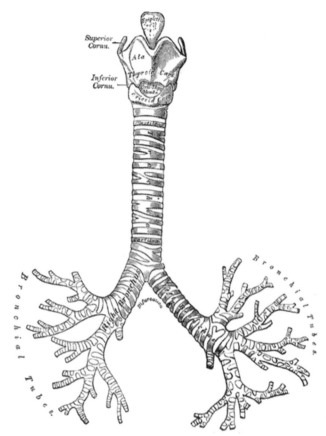

Fig. 46 Fractal geometry of the bronchial tree

perfectly horizontal you will see a symmetrical plain scattered with circular structures. Of course in real life the organs are not perfectly symmetrical and the pathologist's cut is not perfectly horizontal to the central tubes of the system. In fact when you examine the breast carefully you will find up to about 12 ducts opening at the nipple. Each of these is the mouth of a tree-like system for gathering milk at lactation from the glandular elements (lobules) at the terminal ends of the system that look a little like the florets on the surface of broccoli. You can now picture what normal breast tissue looks like under the microscope. It will appear as a collection of circles of varying diameter or as ellipses where the tubule has been cut obliquely. You will also see clusters of tightly packed cells representing the glandular elements that secrete milk. Sometimes you will even spot a tiny terminal tubule emerging from the lobule itself. In addition there will be a lot going on in the spaces between the duct/glandular systems, known as the stroma. In a postmenopausal woman this is mostly fat with scattered blood vessels but in a younger woman it is much more busy. There will be fibrous tissue that acts as a supportive skeleton that stretches and weakens with each pregnancy and lactation or when the glandular structure is replaced with fat. You will also note wandering white cells, scars from earlier episodes of inflammation.

If you then increase the power of the magnification you can look at the detail of the individual tubular structures. In health they are quite banal: one layer of simple cuboidal duct epithelial cells surrounded by a single layer of spindle shaped myo-epithelial cells that are involved in expressing the milk by squeezing it along the tubules. The lobular elements just look like the same cells packed in a parcel. It is remarkable how much havoc these rather boring-looking little blighters cause. (Figure 47)

Next let's increase the power of the simple light microscope to its highest magnification and then we start seeing something of the extraordinary internal organization of these simple-looking cells. In the same way most folk on trying to contemplate the magnitude of

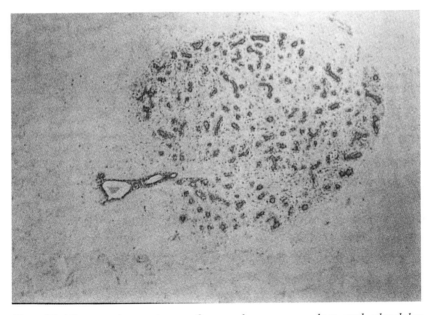

Fig. 47 Microscopic anatomy of normal mammary duct and glandular tissue

outer space and the expanding universe feel giddy with the effort, so I feel giddy whenever I try to contemplate the miraculous miniaturization at the other extreme of the microcosm. The most prominent structure is the nucleus that in health is nice and round and pretty central. This floats in a gooey sea of cytoplasm that also suspends the mitochondria that stoke up the energy to keep this micro-system going. Almost invisible without special staining are the filaments of an endoskeleton that maintains the cell's shape and other fine structures that are cobbling together proteins following the blueprints of the RNA exuded from the nucleus. In the cells of the lobules these proteins contribute to the make-up of milk. The cell is enclosed by a membrane that looks simplicity itself until you have to start envisaging the comings and goings of molecules and the recognitions of chemical signals by specific receptors on the cell surface that alerts the interior mechanisms to either speed up or slow down. Beyond all that and even beyond the highest magnification of the electron microscope we have to try and imagine what's going on at the molecular level. Critics of modern medicine often complain that we practitioners are reductionists who deconstruct the human subject to a molecular level, leaving the person behind. I would argue that in order to fully appreciate this miracle of creation, sensate Homosapiens, with the sense of awe it deserves, we need to be able to **de**construct to a molecular level and then **re**construct upwards through many hierarchical levels to the person living in a family unit within a culture within society. In order to clarify what I mean I will need a short diversion to explain what I believe is the meaning of "holistic medicine".

The English language has a rich and beautiful vocabulary. My Oxford English Dictionary weighs several kilograms and occupies a whole shelf on my bookcase. All these wonderful words have precise meanings. It saddens me to witness how English words are being debased by a pop-culture that encourages transient values and transient meanings to our vocabulary.

Two small examples that I find intensely irritating are the modern usage of the words 'clinical' and 'organic'. Clinical is now used to imply a dispassionate and heartless approach to a subject where the opposite is true in that a good clinician in medical tradition is taken to mean the wise and compassionate elder. Organic, a word with precise meaning in chemistry describing substances whose building blocks are hydrocarbons, is now a slippery word conveying a vague notion of "that which is ecologically sound". The same worry concerns the use of the word holistic when applied to the practice of medicine. Jan Smuts coined the word 'holism' in 1926 and used the word to describe the tendency in nature to produce wholes from the ordered grouping of units. The philosopher and author Arthur Koestler developed the idea more fully in his seminal book 'Janus: A Summing-Up', in which he talks about self-regulating open hierarchic order (SOHO). 'Biological holons are self-regulating open systems which display both the autonomous properties of wholes and the dependent properties of parts. This dichotomy is present on every level of every type of hierarchical organisation and is referred to as the Janus Phenomenon' (Janus is the Roman God that looked in both directions at the same time). Chambers 20th Century Dictionary describes holism in a precise and economical way as follows: 'Complete and self-contained systems from the atom and the cell by evolution to the most complex forms of life and mind'.

It can be seen that the concept of holism is complex and exquisite, and as an open system lends itself to study and experimentation. To do justice to General Jan Smuts' definition of the word holism, we have to start with a reductionist approach to the molecular level, and then from these basic building blocks attempt to reconstruct the complex organism which is the human subject living in harmony within the complex structure of a modern democratic nation state. Since Watson and Crick described the structure and function of DNA in 1953, the development of biological holism has grown way beyond anything Jan Smuts might have envisaged. The basic building block of life has to be a sequence of DNA that codes for a specific protein. These DNA sequences or genes are organised within chromosomes forming the human genome. The chromosomes are packed within the nucleus with an awe-inspiring degree of miniaturisation. The nucleus is a holon looking inwards at the genome and outwards at the cytoplasm of the cell. The cell is a holon that looks inwards at the proteins which guarantee its structure and function contained within its plasma membrane, and at the energy transduction pathways contained within the mitochondria which produce the fuel for life. As a holon, the cell looks outwards at neighbouring cells of a self-similar type which may group together as glandular elements, but the cellular holon also enjoys cross-talk with cells of a different developmental origin communicating by touch through tight junctions, or by the exchange of chemical messages via short-lived paracrine polypeptides. These glandular elements and stromal elements group together as a functioning organ which is holistic in looking inwards at the exquisite functional integrity of itself, and outwards to act in concert with the other organs of the body. This concert is orchestrated at the next level in the holistic hierarchy through the neuro-endocrine/ immunological control mediated via the hypothalamic pituitary axis, the thyroid gland, the adrenal gland, the endocrine glands of sexual identity, and the lympho-reticular system that can distinguish self from non-self. Even this notion of selfness is primitive compared with the next level up the hierarchy where the person exists in a conscious state somewhere within the cerebral cortex, with the mind, the great-unexplored frontier, which will be the scientific challenge of doctors in the new millennium. (Figure 48)

Having got that off my chest you can begin to understand the wonder and respect for creation we experience when looking at a cluster of cells on a slide. With the normal breast cell we begin to imagine "switches" on the cell surface that are ON or OFF. When ON, a signal travels through the cytoplasm to the nucleus to kick-start the process of replication. When the organ recognizes (in some as yet incompletely explained way) that there are enough cells to function properly the switch is turned to OFF. We can also imagine

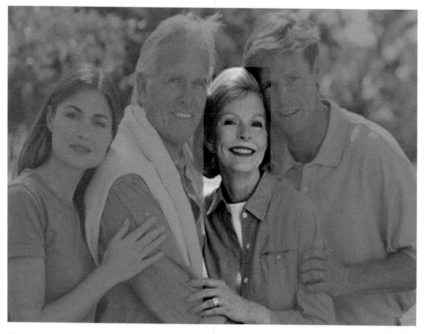

Fig. 48 A woman at the apex of an organized holistic system

the molecules of oestrogen floating through the cell membrane and binding to its receptor. Nowadays of course we can actually visualize the receptors as they stain up nice and brown with a special dye linked to the mono-clonal antibody that homes in on the ER protein. We can then imagine the complex of the hormone and its receptor binding to the precise site on the precise chromosome that triggers the precise menu of proteins that will allow the cell to grow and replicate. Furthermore in preparing for lactation the whole orchestra of the endocrine system bursts into a symphony whereby prolactin secreted from the pituitary gland at the base of the brain ultimately leads to the synthesis of milk proteins from the florets of glandular tissue at the tips of the arborisation of the mammary gland.

The fact that such a complex and beautiful system retains its integrity is the miracle; the fact that some trivial molecular mismanagement can cause the whole system to crash, leading to the death of its host, should not be a surprise.

With all that in mind let me reconstruct the cancer upwards through this hierarchy from the molecule to the metastasis that is the arbiter of a premature death. It is highly probable that all cancers are triggered by acquired genetic defects. Of course it is now well recognized that there are a relatively rare number of families who inherit a breast cancer pre-disposition gene via an inherited germ-line mutation rather than the common "somatic" mutation, but that subject will be covered in the next chapter.

In one way or another this faulty gene leads to the destabilization of the whole of the nuclear apparatus. Morphologically this is seen as the nuclei expand in size and stain darker in colour. They may even become giant cells with a duplication or triplication of the number of chromosomes. To begin with these abnormal cells are constrained within the ducts or lobules where they are described as duct carcinoma in situ (DCIS) or lobular carcinoma in situ (LCIS). Both of these conditions have an unpredictable natural history which perhaps suggests that they are latent pathologies associated with a risk of cancer rather than as obligate pre-cursors. DCIS has another very important property. In many cases the cells lining the duct die off and the cellular debris calcifies. As a result of this these impalpable lesions often show up on mammograms as fine branching calcifications that are diagnosed on screening. Another curious phenomenon is the fact that DCIS appear as multi-focal pathology scattered across the breast in up to 40% of cases. This inevitably leads to a mastectomy. Yet invasive cancers are rarely multifocal. This therefore has to

157

imply that once a focus of DCIS decides to become invasive all the other foci are either suppressed by the invasive component or simply regress naturally. The paradox therefore is that a woman is just as likely to suffer a mastectomy for DCIS ("very early" cancer) as for the invasive disease. I will return to this matter in chapter 19. Eventually a proportion of these pre-cursor (latent) cancer cells change functionally. They literally lose their inhibitions, replicate rapidly and feel free to seek new pastures by wandering off to seek fertile new soil well away from their native land. This process is expedited by their new ability to infiltrate capillaries of the vascular and lymphatic system for random dissemination anywhere in the body to form metastases. The cells become disinhibited in other weird ways as well. Most mature cells shut down most of their genome, so that only the genes needed to survive and function in health are active. Yet we must remember that all cells in the adult body contain within their nucleus the blueprints for any other phenotype (progeny) of cell in any other organ in the body. Rarely in breast cancer we see this process reversed so that the breast cells take on the appearance of squamous cells (spindle shaped), muscle cells or even cartilage. This process is called metaplasia. Most of the time it is ignored but I find it fascinating. It tends to be associated with a grave prognosis. Along with all this ugliness, the duct and lobular epithelium lose their fractal geometry I described earlier.

In our multi-disciplinary meetings, as well as confirming the diagnosis we also try and calculate the prognosis and plan rational therapy. The prognosis is literally in direct proportion to the ugliness of what we see. (Figure 49) If the cells still look a little like breast cells and if ductular structures can still be made out, then that is a grade I cancer with a good prognosis. If the cells look like nothing on earth and there is nothing left of the tubular structures, then that is a grade III tumour with a poor prognosis. In between of course we have the grade II cancers. The evidence of free cancer cells in the vascular or lymphatic channels also estimates prognosis and the number of lymph nodes invaded by cancer is also directly proportional to the outcome. The presence or absence of the hormone receptors not only allows planning for endocrine therapy but is also a prognostic index. The same applies to the HER 2 status of the tumour. HER2 positive tumours tend to relapse early but also have the advantage of responding dramatically to *herceptin.*

Armed with all these data together with the Xray, ultrasound and scanning information, the school of Athens is then in a position

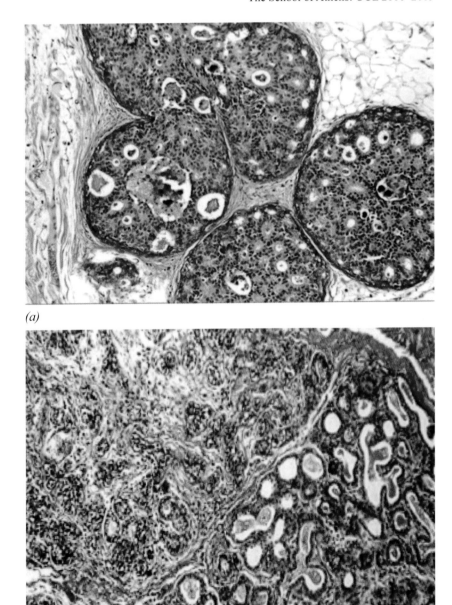

(a)

(b)

Fig. 49 a) Duct carcinoma in situ b) The disorganized microscopic anatomy of a grade III invasive breast cancer adjacent to an area of DCIS

for making informed and rational programmes of treatment for the individual patients. This kind of teamwork alone has improved outcomes over the last decade or two and I am proud to have shared the company of so many wise and compassionate friends and colleagues.

****

At the end of the weekly MDM, round about 09.00am, I would leave the Rockefeller building at UCH and resume my odyssey to the Elizabeth Garret Anderson (EGA) hospital in order to confront my patients with the esoteric secrets of their disease revealed by the microscope and our new knowledge of molecular biology. I would turn north up Gower Street walking in front of the massive cupola emblematic of University College London and then nip down Gower Place, running eastward along by the service entrances to the university. I always looked out for two men in blue coveralls who would be talking in an animated way about the latest football scores using the sign language of the deaf. For some reason this sight would lift my spirits. Crossing into Endsleigh Gardens I would always pause outside the Quaker Friends House assembly rooms. I love the Quakers, they have no extreme group of fundamentalists and all of them are equal in the sight of the Lord. Here, just before you encounter the roar of the Euston Road, is a peaceful oasis of a rose garden. In the summer when the blooms are at their best I would enjoy another boost to my sense of well being before taking my life in my hands in negotiating the complexities of crossing six lanes of traffic with frustrated London drivers jumping the lights.

Finally down a quiet side street behind the fire station I would come to the EGA. I loved the EGA. It was small and fit for the purpose of serving the needs of women's health. The Elizabeth Garret Anderson was named after its founder, the first female medical graduate in Europe, whose formidable and tightly corseted sepia image welcomed you on entering the lobby. Not long after I retired from the NHS this wonderful little hospital was sold off as part of the private funding initiative (PFI) to help pay for the new, state of the art University College Hospital that dominates the block along the Euston Road between Gower Street and Tottenham Court Road.

Girding my loins I would then climb three flights of stairs to the breast clinic.

This area of London is truly multicultural and multi-ethnic, as reflected in the skin colours and exotic costumes of the women waiting to be registered. Walking through the waiting room I would smile at old friends and note the body language of strangers. Some would carry away good news that their tumour was purely in situ and carried an almost 100% chance of cure. Others would bear the burden of the bad news that their tumour was high grade, ER negative and with multiple lymph nodes involved. They would have to endure six months of chemotherapy and six weeks of radiotherapy and yet still have to live with the uncertainty that the disease could strike again any time in the future. The courage of these women was phenomenal. They seemed more concerned about how their family might take it than themselves, and on each subsequent visit asked after my health before I had a chance to ask after theirs. No wonder my wife and daughters often had to suffer short shrift from me after such days. Judy, bless her, soon learnt to have a bottle of my favourite malt whisky to hand at 6.00pm on a Tuesday evening, before debriefing began.

Chapter 14

The Proband's Tale*

My son-in-law is a "Cohen" and I am proud of the fact that my daughter has married into this princely and scholarly lineage. My son-in-law's father is Rabbi Dr Jeffrey Cohen and through the oral tradition they can trace their roots back to the Cohenim (Tribe of Priests) of the Temple in Jerusalem. We now know that this oral tradition has been scientifically confirmed by studying the Y chromosome of Cohenim. The Y chromosome is associated with the male sex and handed down through the generations from father to son. The Y chromosome of the Cohenim has certain characteristics that are common to all the Cohenim in the world, confirming the veracity of the oral tradition.

Perhaps more remarkable and certainly more relevant to this book is the tradition that our Jewish ethnicity is handed down through the maternal line. Every cell in the human body has two sources of DNA. The major source is within the nucleus and this can be described as the blueprint that codifies our personhood, in other words the way we look, our height, the colour of our eyes and to a large extent our attitudes and intelligence.

Hidden in the cytoplasm between the nucleus and the cell membrane and only clearly seen under electron microscopy are the mitochondria. These tiny structures are vitally important in burning food in order to provide the energy for cellular activity. In other words they are operating as power stations at the molecular level.

*A person who has some distinctive characteristic and who serves as a starting point for a genetic study of the transmission of this feature.

The mitochondria are peculiar. Way back in the very early days in the evolution of living organisms, there was once a tribe of primitive "bacteria", that appeared to have made a pact of mutual self interest whereby the primitive cell would provide the primitive "bacteria" succour and protection in return for them to take over the task of providing green energy. This remarkable symbiosis can be judged by the fact that eons later these saprophytes (facultative parasites) still retain some of their own original DNA that codes for a few proteins that are essential for the organization of these "organelles". This mitochondrial DNA is now known to be entirely maternal in origin, handed down through the generations via the female line. The reason for this is simple. The ovum has many mitochondria, whereas the sperm is essentially a motorized packet of nuclear DNA. So the mitochondrial DNA in the fertilized egg is all maternal. As is the case for the Y chromosome, mitochondrial DNA also differs in subtle detail between individuals, and through this it is possible to trace the origins and migration of peoples of different ethnicity from the first hominids who evolved from the apes in Central Africa in the dark distant past. Once again genetic anthropology confirms that the majority of people who consider themselves Jewish are indeed Jewish as judged by their mitochondrial DNA. Subtle differences in this coding also allows us to trace the migration of the Jewish people over time and even suggests that our origins might indeed have arisen from four different matriarchal tribes.

Sadly along the way the Jewish people have collected a number of deleterious mutations within the cellular DNA of the germ line that has also been passed on through the generations. These include the mutations that are associated with Tay Sachs disease as well the BRCA mutations that increase the risk of developing breast cancer. The origin of these mutations in time can be traced by considering the migration and dispersion of the Jewish people in ancient history. The story starts about 3000 years ago.

In 586BC following the Babylonian conquest and the fall of the first Temple the major Jewish dispersion was to Mesopotamia; "by the rivers of Babylon, there we set down, yea we wept when we remembered Zion" (Psalm 137). Some Jews migrated to Egypt and others North into Syria. After the passage of years many Jews drifted back to the land of Israel but after the revolt against Persia, 359–338BC, many Jews migrated north towards the Caspian Sea with gradual migrations through trading further north into Europe. The Jews who migrated to Mesopotamia enjoyed a long history emerging ultimately as Iraqi Jews, all of whom were expelled after the Second World War.

The next cataclysmic event in Jewish history was the sacking of the second Temple by the Romans in 70CE. This event was celebrated by the Roman legions in the bas-relief seen on the arch of Titus in Rome, where the Temple menorah is seen carried on the shoulders of the triumphal Roman legionnaires. This is also celebrated by the coin that was struck embossed with the words Judea Capta. (Figure 50) At this point 80,000 Jewish slaves were shipped across to the Roman province of Hispania and settled in the region just south of Cordoba. This colony ultimately gave rise to the Sephardic population. Some Jews remained behind in cities such as Jerusalem, Hebron and S'fad with descendents to this very day, whereas others continued their migration through Asia Minor into Eastern Europe. Until the expulsion of the Jews from Portugal and Spain at the end of the 15th Century, there was very little inter-marriage between the Sephardim and the Jews in Mesopotamia, Asia Minor and Europe. With these historical facts in mind it is then all the more interesting to look at the distribution of the BRCA 1 and BRCA 2 mutations amongst women from the different Jewish communities.

To put it into perspective, mutation within these genes in the majority of populations occur with a frequency of between 1 in 300 and 1 in 800. The second highest frequency is seen in Iceland where about 1 in 170 (0.6%) of women are affected. However amongst Jewish women within Israel 1 in 40 women (2.5%) are affected and then when you look at the individual genes you see how the history of the Jewish

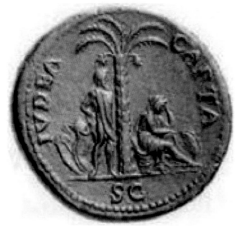

Fig. 50 Roman coin engraved with Judea Capta, circa 70 CE

people has been reflected, once again at the molecular level. First of all Sephardi women do not carry any of these mutations. Therefore the mutations that have been identified must have occurred after the fall of the second Temple or amongst those families who remained in Mesopotamia or migrated north after the fall of the first Temple. There are three "Jewish" mutations. These can be roughly dated by analysis of mitochondrial DNA. The oldest mutation (185del AG) on the BRCA 1 gene occurs in 1% of both Ashkenazi and Iraqi Jews and is estimated to be between two and a half and three thousand years old. This therefore must have occurred by a founder germ line mutation in Mesopotamia shortly after the fall of the first Temple and also have been carried north amongst those Jews who ultimately contributed to the foundation of the Ashkenazi tribes.

The second mutation (617del IT) is on the BRCA 2 gene and is found in 1.4% of Ashkenazi Jews only and is estimated to be about 700 years old. Clearly long after the fall of the second Temple and almost certainly the founder germ line mutation, it must have arisen from the Jews who had settled in Eastern Europe. The third mutation (5382ins C) is on the BRCA 1 gene and occurs in 0.1% of the Jewish population and is said to reflect another tragic event in Jewish history. This mutation is also seen amongst high-risk non-Jewish women of Eastern European origin and is sometimes described as a "pogrom" mutation. In other words the consequence of pregnancies following rape, yet another component in the repertoire of humiliations experienced in the Jewish ghettos of the Pale of Settlement between the 13th and 19th centuries.

These three BRCA mutations are distributed amongst Jewish people in an identical way in New York and Manchester. The incidence and type of mutations amongst the Manchester Ashkenazi population has been documented and described by Professor Gareth Evans. Both the Israeli and the British experience confirm that women carrying one of the BRCA 1 mutations have a close on 80% chance of developing breast cancer by the time they are 80, whereas those carrying the BRCA 2 mutations have about a 35% chance of developing breast cancer by the age of 80. These mutations are also associated for an increased risk of ovarian cancer but also, curiously enough, prostate cancer, amongst the male members of the family. Rarely can these mutations be carried and express themselves as breast cancer in the male relatives of such at risk groups.

The experience of all the workers in this field has confirmed that what marks these cancers out as a uniquely difficult problem is the early age of onset, which is on average ten to fifteen years younger than what you might expect with sporadic breast cancer. For that reason they occur more often in pre-menopausal women where mammography is singularly unhelpful. The other curiosity about these cancers is their morphology (how they look under a microscope) and the increasing understanding of why these specific mutations contribute to an early presentation with the disease. Professor Alan Ashworth, the Head of Breakthrough Breast Cancer at the Institute of Cancer Research in London has explained the biology of these cancers. It appears that the normal BRCA genes have a central role in the repair of DNA. The DNA in our body is constantly being damaged either spontaneously at the time of cell division (transcription error) or by exogenous factors such as ambient radiation or cosmic rays. For those with a deep understanding of the subject the miracle isn't why people get cancer but how the species survives at all, *free of cancer*. Clearly, a long way back in the evolution of mankind, a necessary condition for life was the development of extremely rapid DNA repair systems. Thousands of mutations occur in our body daily and these are closely monitored and repaired with mechanisms of awe-inspiring ingenuity that makes one speculate about "intelligent design". The BRCA mutations mean that these repair mechanisms are disturbed, and if a number of these DNA fractures or faults of transcription are allowed to accumulate, then the cell takes on the malignant potential of unchecked cellular division and dissemination.

****

So what, if anything, can be done about those unfortunate families? For the moment there are two possibilities to consider, firstly prophylactic mastectomy (with or without prophylactic oophorectomy) and secondly pre-implantation embryo selection. I look upon this prophylactic mastectomy as a barbaric but perhaps necessary "intermediate" technology. In other words trying to make the least bad decision when options are few and far between.

In 1996 whilst working at the Royal Marsden Hospital I had to face this problem for the first time shortly after the BRCA1 gene was identified, and record this experience in a paper entitled "The Proband's tale", with the help of Dr. Ros Eeles, a brilliant clinical geneticist who combines an understanding of the esoterica of molecular biology with a kind and sensitive approach to the subject and her family. In this publication we concluded that the identification of the BRCA1 gene might prove a mixed blessing in the short term. First, the demand for testing might outstrip available resources, the ethics of testing are complex and the advice to give someone who tests positive were as yet unclear. Furthermore, the psychological dynamics within such families had not yet been considered seriously. As these families might be widespread, there will inevitably be problems involving clinical genetic centres in different parts of the country, or for that matter, in different areas of the world. In the paper we provided a case report, which might have been considered as an adumbration of things to come. The proband in this story (a co-author) was known to have inherited a genetic predisposition to cancer. This was because her identical twin had already developed the disease and she came from a kindred with a very high probability for carrying a dominant breast cancer gene in the germ line. We described the personal reactions of an individual woman faced with these difficult decisions, the impact on her family and the impact on the clinical genetic services in different parts of the country. Our experience helped to provide a template for the development of regional services once genetic testing for predisposition to breast cancer became widely available. After exhaustive counselling "the proband" agreed that I should proceed with removing both her breasts prophylactically with implants to replace their volume. In a way I could almost claim to have done the first prophylactic mastectomy for a BRCA1 carrier in the UK just before the test became routinely available. I have a sense of shame rather than pride about this ignoble "first", there must be better ways, soon to be discovered, of handling the problem. In the meantime if that isn't bad enough, women of today presenting with a breast cancer diagnosis and then discovered to be carrying mutant BRCA 1/2 genes also have to face a tough decision on whether or not to have the other breast removed as well as the ovaries. Approximately 50% of such women are accepting these mutilations in a desperate attempt of reducing their chances of another cancer whilst still at hazard from their first. This is the cruellest dilemma one can imagine for a young woman to face.

On Wednesday the 10th of May 2007, the British Human Fertilisation and Embryology Authority (HFEA) gave the go ahead for pre-implantation genetic diagnosis for the selection of embryos free of the mutations that predispose to breast or colo-rectal cancer. The hysterical overreaction of some sections of the press and the television studios was predictable. On the one hand we had the shrill warnings that this was the slippery slope to "Eugenics" and on the other hand we had members of affected families saying that the decision was a "no brainer". Let me deal first of all with this reaction quickly before getting bogged down in what is a very complex ethical biomedical debate.

The tiresome morsel of American jargon, "no brainer", has slipped into common English usage quite recently and appears to have been adopted by those who have no valid opinions of their own. I suppose it stands in for "that which is self-evident", amongst English speaking people. I heard it used in a television interview with a woman in her early forties, carrying a BRCA1 mutation, a member of an extended family with a strong family history of breast and ovarian cancer. What I found so grotesque about that statement apart from the mutilation of my mother tongue, was the fact that if PGD had been available one generation earlier, she would not have been here to offer up her opinion. She might indeed have the right, after extensive counselling, to decide for herself to go through the rigours and expense of IVF and PGD, but to suggest that the rightness of that decision was self-evident trivialises the issue.

Now let us try and get to grips with slippery slopes and eugenics. The term "eugenics" was coined by Francis Galton (1822–1911). He was an English scientist who studied heredity and intelligence and happened to be a cousin of Charles Darwin. Erasmus Darwin was Francis Galton's maternal grandfather and also Charles Darwin's paternal grandfather, so Galton was indeed fortunate to have been born into a family whose genetic pool included members of the Wedgwood and Keynes families. Galton defined his new word this way: "Eugenics is the study of agencies under social control that may improve or impair the racial qualities of future generations, whether physically or mentally." He described the three stages of eugenics, first an academic matter, then a practical policy, and finally that "it must be introduced into the national consciousness as a new religion." He elaborated on his ideas in an article entitled "Hereditary Character and Talent" (published in two parts in *MacMillan's Magazine,* vol. 11, November 1864 and April 1865, pp. 157–166, 318–327), expressing his frustration that no one was breeding a better human race:

"If a twentieth part of the cost and pains were spent in measures for the improvement of the human race that is spent on the improvement of the breed of horses and cattle, what a galaxy of genius might we not create! We might introduce prophets and high priests of civilization into the world, as surely as we

*can propagate idiots by mating cretins. Men and women of the
present day are, to those we might hope to bring into existence,
what the pariah dogs of the streets of an Eastern town are to
our own highly-bred varieties."*

What is so chilling about reading these ramblings of an old Victorian
bigot one hundred years later is the fact that Adolf Hitler and the
Third Reich attempted to apply these principles in practice with mass
sterilisation of inmates of mental asylums and undesirable non-Aryans
as a prelude to mass murder.

I'm pretty sure that the HFEA does not have in mind that we should
start building a master race of blond, blue eyed, athletic geniuses, but
is their endorsement of PGD to select out embryos predetermined
to develop cancer in young adulthood the first step down a slippery
slope towards a Galtonian Utopia? I think not. For a start I don't
subscribe to the "slippery slope" principle in ethics debates. This
presupposes that there is a line of ethical principle that must never
be crossed that is viewed from a point on the moral high ground. One
step down, one concession, one turning of a blind eye and society
loses its footing sliding downwards into the ethical abyss. This as you
see is argument by analogy. We have already made concessions in
selecting babies. For example amniocentesis is commonly used before
aborting foetuses with X linked haemophilia or Downs' syndrome.
This technique can be abused for sex selection but such abuse is
covered by law. A recent high-profile case in India ended when a
gynaecologist who profited by aborting female foetuses was given
a stiff jail sentence. No doubt the problem is rife in China where
there is a one-child policy, but in this example sex selection is the
consequence of social engineering, not the reverse.

Furthermore PGD is already available for families bearing the
gene for cystic fibrosis, Tay Sachs disease, Huntingdon's chorea and
thalassaemia; all dreadful diseases with early age onset. This as far
as I know has never been associated with a slide down the slope of
ethical compromise. So what makes the new ruling so controversial?
In screening embryos for the BRCA mutations that predispose to
breast cancer the word is predispose. In other words not inevitable.
For example BRCA2 has about a 50% penetrance for breast cancer
and breast cancer can be prevented by prophylactic mastectomy for
all cases with BRCA mutations. These are not trivial interventions
but have to be weighed up against the very nature of personhood. I
can see how PGD could breed out the faulty gene in the fullness of

time and spare mothers from the guilt and anxiety of passing it on, but I can also understand the argument that you might be destroying an embryo, albeit only eight cells in total, that might lead to an adult of unknown potential who might lead a full and productive life. At the same time I know that left to nature about half such embryos at this stage of gestation would spontaneously abort, or as Gillian Lockwood, chairman of the British Fertility Society's ethical committee so eloquently put it; "half the eggs fertilised naturally don't become babies and we are not in a perpetual state of mourning". So can I take a position on this? Well like all of us it's only when it's up front and personal that the hypothetical debate becomes a matter of serious decision-making.

As I described in the preface to this book our family went through a period of crisis when my sister agreed to be tested for a BRCA mutation because of the familial pre-disposition to breast cancer, for the sake of her four daughters. Fortunately she (and by inference my nieces) tested negative. Had she tested positive I don't think I would have wanted the gene bred out of the family because I'm confident that in such cases breast cancer will one day be preventable and in due course curable. Furthermore for all we know breeding out one undesirable gene might be associated with the inadvertent loss of a desirable gene from the same pool.

Those are my opinions but in the end the technology is here to stay, it cannot be un-invented, and like all technology can be used for good or for evil. What is needed is control and mature debate. It's neither eugenics nor a no brainer.

Chapter 15

The Golden Ibex of Santorini

3,600 years ago the Greek island of Santorini (Thera) blew its top. In the most cataclysmic volcanic eruption in the recorded history of our planet, 30 cubic kms of magma in the form of pumice and volcanic ash buried the island and its civilisation. These dramatic events have given rise to a number of legends and myths. Firstly the destroyed civilisation of the island of Strongili (as the island was known before the eruption) gave rise to the legend of the lost city of Atlantis. The apparent sudden destruction of the Minoan civilisation on the island of Crete has been ascribed to this catastrophic event and the tidal wave that followed in its wake. Finally the timing of the volcanic eruption was undoubtedly close to the timing of the exodus of the Jews from ancient Egypt and a rational explanation for the ten plagues described in the Old Testament. Some of the predicted events with a volcanic eruption of this magnitude might account for the plagues. For example the column of ash above the volcano could produce a shadow long enough for the sun to be obliterated at noon over ancient Egypt. Furthermore the inflow of the Mediterranean Sea into the volcanic cavity, followed by the mighty tidal wave or tsunami, might have accounted for the dry crossing of the *Reed* Sea (probably the Nile delta rather than the Red Sea as known today) by Moses and the children of Israel, followed by the destruction of Pharaoh and his legions, shortly thereafter. Bible stories and legends of lost civilisations are romantic but the reality might exceed the expectations of many sceptics. (Figure 51)

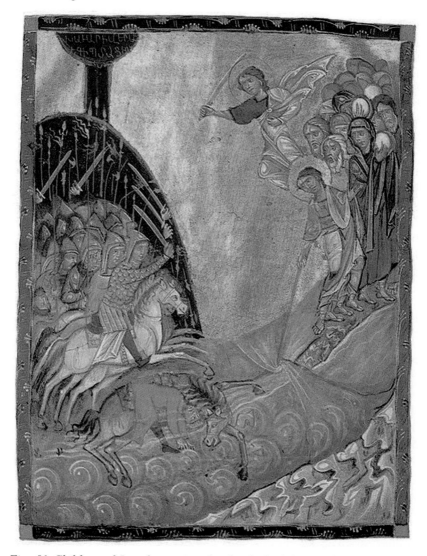

Fig. 51 Children of Israel crossing the dry bed of the Reed Sea before the tsunami triggered by the eruption of the volcanic island of Strongili, circa 1,500 BCE

Approximately ten years ago a shaft was being dug to provide foundations for a permanent protective cover over the archaeological excavations at Akrotiri, a site at the southern tip of the crescent shaped island. Amongst the rubble, a workman discovered a perfectly preserved wooden box that was thought to serve some late bronze-age domestic role. On opening the box, the archaeologists were astonished to discover a most beautifully crafted and perfectly preserved Golden Ibex about the size of a new born kitten. Closer inspection revealed that it was hollow with all four limbs welded at the junction with the trunk. The local experts assumed it was fabricated by using the lost wax technique but the technique for welding the limbs onto the trunk was a mystery; as was its role within this lost civilisation (Figure 52)

As an object this sublimely proportioned artefact can be looked upon in three ways. Firstly as an object venerated for its beauty and, for all we know, venerated in its time as a household God, a pocket size representation of the Golden Calf worshipped by the children of Israel a few years after the exodus from Egypt. Secondly it could be looked upon as an archaeological curiosity capable of throwing light on the bronze-age civilisations of the Cicladean Islands and their trading links with ancient Egypt to the south and the biblical kingdoms to the east. Finally it was a technological challenge to assay the gold and interpret the technique for joining the limbs to the trunk without damaging the find that in its own way would shed light on its archaeological provenance.

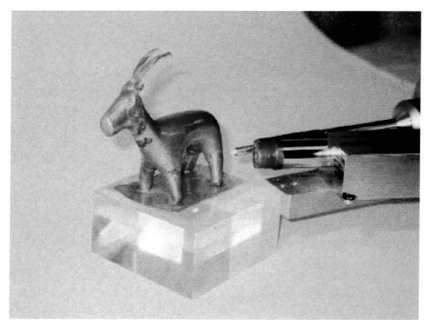

Fig. 52 The Golden Ibex of Santorini

In the last week of August 1997, a group of us assembled on Santorini as guests of Mr Peter Nomikos, the founder of Photoelectron Corporation, for a scientific advisory board meeting. I had been working with Photoelectron Corporation for about three years developing a technique for intra-operative radiotherapy in the treatment of early breast cancer using a miniature X-ray generating source developed by the company. This device, about the size and the shape of a woman's handbag, accelerates electrons down a metallic capillary tube which then hit a gold target generating soft X-rays from a point source at its tip. Introduced within the cavity following wide local excision of an early breast cancer it can deliver a full booster dose of radiation to the excision margins; I'll expand on this shortly. The Nomikos Foundation also supports the archaeological explorations of Akrotiri and for that reason I was privileged to witness an historic first in the history of archaeology.

On Sunday 31st August, a group consisting of archaeologists, technologists and oncologists gathered in the subterranean laboratories of the archaeological museum in Thera. Also in our number was the great pianist and conductor Vladimir Ashkenasi, another house guest of the Nomikos family. The Golden Ibex was placed upon a laboratory table and the miniature X-ray source was directed precisely at the weld at the junction between a hind limb and the trunk of this enigmatic beast. The device was switched on, electrons were accelerated down the capillary tube and X-rays from the gold target at the tip of the device excited the molecules within the Bronze Age weld of the ancient gold of the Ibex. The signal from the excitation of these molecules was then picked up by another extraordinary technological invention developed for the NASA Mars exploration project. This detection probe then provided us with a wave-form printout describing the precise content of the solder. Thus with the benefits of modern technology the artisan of an ancient Cicladean culture was able to speak to us over the centuries. It is difficult to describe the sense of wonder we all experienced at this unique amalgam of art, archaeology and technology. The results from this experiment were quite remarkable and confirmed that the artisan was a visitor from the second millennium BC Ancient Egypt and the Golden Ibex was buried at the time of the biblical exodus from Egypt. To think that I handled a household god manufactured by a similar technique and within a few years of the golden calf at the foot of Mount Sinai still makes my hair prickle on the back of my neck. Shortly after that experiment we all retired to the Nomikos castle for a celebratory drink only to learn of the tragic death of Princess Diana in an underpass in Paris.

So how did all this come about and what is the relevance to the treatment of breast cancer? One of the undoubted charms of research is the making of connections from random observations often from disciplines other than your own. Another useful asset is the gift of serendipidity. Two events collided that have lead to a very important breakthrough in the management of breast cancer. One personified by Peter Nomikos and the other personified by Jaynant Vaidya. Peter is the doyen of a great Greek shipping family. Peter is charming, elegant and aristocratic. His beautiful wife Dola shares the same qualities. Between them they own most of the land on Santorini and enjoy a friendly competition in the production of fine white wines. Personally I think Mrs. Nomikos' wines are better but don't tell Peter. They own the castle and its complex of pools, gardens and habitable caves that dominates the skyline visible as the cruise ships enter the harbour. This golden couple's life was blighted by the loss of one of their children at the age of 11 from a virulent form of cancer, and Peter always wanted to give something back to the oncology community as a fitting memorial for their son. Peter also owned a small high-tech company in the USA. His physicists invented a miniature electron generator and found themselves with "a technology for which there was no known disease", although in fairness their original idea was to use it in the stereotactic treatment of brain tumours. As I had treated one of their friends for breast cancer Peter and his physicist came to visit me shortly after I was appointed to the chair in surgery at University College London in 1995. The challenge they offered was to use the technology for the management of early breast cancer.

In parallel with all this, another interesting character entered my sphere of influence. About a year before this started, my old friend Indraneel (Neel) Mittra, the head of the breast cancer centre at the Tata Memorial Hospital Mumbai, asked me to take a look at one of his post graduate students, Mr. Jayant (Jay) Vaidya, who he claimed was one of the brightest young medical graduates in the whole of India. Neel thought that I might find it worthwhile to take him on as a PhD student. My first impressions of Jay were not auspicious. He wore a shapeless suit, the scruffiest of shoes and spoke with an almost impenetrable Indian accent. However it didn't take long to learn that in his own way he was a bit of an aristocrat. The name Vaidya describes his origins from a long line of traditional ayurvedic healers, his grandfather is honoured with a statue in the central square of Goa and his late and lamented father, a public health doctor, was a great man who singlehandedly successfully campaigned for making Goa the first tobacco-free state in the world. The next thing I learnt about Jay was his incandescent intelligence. I myself am often described as someone capable of thinking "outside the box". If that is the case then young Jay could out-pace me by thinking into the fourth dimension. One piece of work he had completed in Mumbai shortly before coming to the UK concerned the "multi-focality" of breast cancer. Although by this time the default therapy for early breast cancer was "lumpectomy", it was assumed that following surgery the whole of the breast had to be treated with 6 weeks of post-operative radiotherapy to mop up any occult foci of disease outside the vicinity of the primary cancer. Jay's study involved a careful analysis of several hundred mastectomy specimens, cutting them in 50 thin slices and then mapping out according to three dimensional co-ordinates the number and position of areas of cancer outside the primary focus, that were unsuspected on clinical and radiological grounds. These areas weren't just a few cells but fully formed foci of in-situ or invasive disease below the threshold of size for mammographic detection. Over 60% of breasts had these hidden foci and most of them were well away from the dominant (index) primary. (Most readers would then jump to the conclusion that this was a vindication of the policy of whole breast radiation). And yet, and yet... now we must prepare ourselves for a paradox. After breast-conserving surgery the results of most observational studies or clinical trials have demonstrated that 90% of recurrent disease in the breast after surgery is within the index quadrant in the presence *or absence* of whole breast radiation. This counter-intuitive observation has both biological and clinical consequences. Biologically this tells us that not all that looks like cancer under the microscope will behave like cancer. I choose to call this "latent disease" and will deal with this at length in chapters 18 and 19. The clinical consequence of this observation suggests that maybe we don't have to treat the whole breast but only the immediate area around the tumour bed after removal of the primary. If that is the case then maybe we could complete all the treatment at the time of surgery by irradiating the tumour bed exposed after the removal of the primary disease.

After two years of R & D we had developed a prototype for the first clinical trial. This consisted of a gantry that would hold the device steady in three-dimensional space. In addition we had manufactured for use a selection of applicators with a hollow sphere at the end.

The idea being that the electrons would be accelerated down a metal capillary tube hitting a gold target at its tip. This bombardment would release X-rays that would spread out in a spheroidal configuration. The tip of the tube sat precisely at the epicentre of the spheroidal plastic applicator of a size chosen to fit the cavity after the tumour was excised. This way the walls of the tumour cavity would be irradiated to a very high dose that rapidly attenuated over a distance of a few centimetres, as a result of which the vital organs of the patient would be spared, the operator would be out of harm's way, and the device could be used in any operating theatre without the need of lead shielding. (Figure 53) Anyway that was the theory. A very courageous lady with a small breast cancer volunteered to be the first patient and neither of us had a good night's sleep before the morning of the operation. With my dear friend Jeff Tobias the radiotherapist and his team of physicists standing by and Jay on the other side of the operating table and my heart somewhere close to my epiglottis, I cut out the tumour, stopped the bleeding, chose the

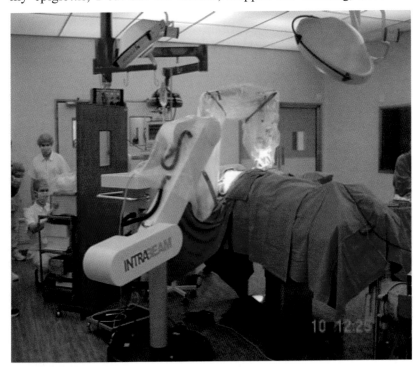

Fig. 53 The INTRABEAM equipment in use for intra-operative radiotherapy

applicator with a sphere that fitted snugly in the cavity, inserted the electron beam tube, turned on the machine and stepped out of the theatre for 25 minutes, leaving the anaesthetist, in theory, out of range. Some times you have to get lucky as well as getting good. As chance would have it the surface of the applicator and the surface of the interior of the breast adhered to each other which meant the geometric conformation of the radiation to the target was perfect. Next, as predicted, the anaesthetist's radiation badge showed no fogging, so he may yet father children, and finally the crude guess at dosimetry proved correct. Of course the latter was only confirmed in the fullness of time, and I'm certainly not going to bore my readers with the esoterica of radiobiology. The next night I couldn't sleep as I considered the implications of this tentative step forward. Meanwhile the patient slept well and made a full and uneventful recovery.

The implications of this leap in the dark are profound. If it works out, then many women will be spared seven weeks of treatment traipsing back and forth to the radiotherapy centre. Furthermore tens of thousands of women in the developing world who live hundreds of miles from a radiotherapy unit, or in countries that can't afford the multi-million pound investment, will be able to enjoy the advantages of breast conservation, by bringing the radiotherapy unit to the patient. Mountains and Mohammed come to mind. In countries like ours the waiting list for post-operative radiotherapy would vanish at a stroke and we estimate the NHS would be saved £15,000,000 a year. So far 300 women have been treated in pilot studies and followed up for five years, without ill effect and with a remarkably low local recurrence rate. We also have a multinational clinical trial of intra-operative radiotherapy alone versus conventional post-operative radiotherapy that has, at the time of writing, recruited about 2,000 patients. 25 collaborating centres are dotted round the world from Europe to California and to southwest Australia. I suspect that by the time this book is published we will have identified groups of women where the one shot of X rays at the time of surgery will be just as effective as the exhausting three to six weeks of conventional treatment. Along the way the radiobiological studies lead by Professor Frederik Wenz of Mannheim University even suggest the novel approach might be better.

Sadly the first casualty of the programme was Photo-electron Corp. that went into receivership. Fortunately the Karl Zeiss Corporation in Germany was able to step in and manufacture what is now known as INTRABEAM. Finally as I retire from clinical practice I am indeed fortunate that Jay Vaidya was ready to take my place, smartly dressed, shoes polished, accent improved and brain as sharp as ever.

The Golden Ibex of Santorini may yet turn out to be an omen of good luck for the thousands of women who will inevitably develop breast cancer in decades to come.

****

As chance would have it shortly after I announced my retirement from clinical practice at the end of May 2009, a favourite Greek patient of mine, Mrs Odette K, together with her ebullient husband George, invited us for a holiday with them at a beautiful resort complex on the island, as a way of thanking me for saving her life. I certainly never claimed to have saved her life but if that was her belief then it would have been churlish to have refused such a generous offer, and as I had retired there was no professional conflict of interest. *("Methinks he doth protest too much")* We met in Athens in mid August that year and flew the short hop to the azure-edged extinct volcano, to take up temporary residence in a glamorous apartment built into the face of the cliff, with breakfast served from a terrace overlooking the caldera. On an impulse we took ourselves off to see if the Nomikos family was at home, accompanied by Mrs. K who was to act as an interpreter to get us past the security perimeter of the high walled compound. Our luck was in because for the first time that year, the family had taken up residence in anticipation of the wedding of their son, Peter (Petros) junior. We hadn't met for at least five years yet Peter senior greeted me like a long lost brother as we emerged breathless at the top of our climb from Fira 300 steep steps below. As we stepped out on their plateau, his wife Dola emerged from the pool like Aphrodite, unchanged in appearance from the last time we were there 10 years earlier, the image of the Greek Goddess portrayed by Botticelli (although with a bobbed hair cut). The three of us were invited to an *al fresco* lunch and their delight at learning how their initiative was about to change the face of breast cancer management knew no bounds. They claimed it was one of the best wedding gifts they could have dreamed of. We made our farewells in good time so as to allow them to change in order to welcome their guest of honour, ex King Constantine of the Hellenes.

Chapter 16

The Illusions and Disillusions of Screening

"The largest threat posed by American medicine is that more and more of us are being drawn into the system not because of an epidemic of disease, but because of an epidemic of diagnoses. The real problem with the epidemic of diagnoses is that it leads to an epidemic of treatments. Not all treatments have important benefits, but almost all can have harms"*

A couple of weeks ago I was showing off my newly acquired iPhone to my very bright 12-year-old granddaughter when she elected to "Google" my name. To my amazement the top hit appeared to link my name with that of Jade Goody. As far as I could recall I had never met with her, I have never knowingly watched "Big Brother," and I don't even research or treat cervical cancer. It appears that I was being stigmatized as the leading anti-screening dinosaur. Everything became clear when on Monday 23rd March 2009 The Times published a full page obituary on the short and tragic life of the reality TV celebrity, Jade Goody, whose dying wish was that women under the age of 25 should have access to screening for cervical cancer. The "Goody effect" has already provoked a campaign and a response from the department of health. I have nothing against the late Jade, in fact she reminded me of the type of patient that used to make my NHS clinics in central London such fun.

*What's Making Us Sick Is an Epidemic of Diagnoses H Gilbert Welch, Lisa Schwartz and Steven Woloshin, The New York Times, January 2, 2007

Nevertheless I feel the urge to defend myself and to explain why being a screening sceptic might after all place me on the side of the angels rather than to the darker side of Darth Vader. For a start I must hasten to mention that some of my best friends are women. As already described my beloved mother died of breast cancer and my equally beloved sister is a long-term survivor of the disease. Galvanized by this experience I've devoted my whole professional life to fighting breast cancer, visualizing it as a slavering beast, and in moments of self-delusion seeing myself as St. Michael. My wife's reminder, that this brand name is sewn in the back of my underpants, tends to bring me down to earth.

In addition I actually know a thing or two about screening. In 1987 when I was employed as Professor of Surgery at King's College Hospital, I was commissioned by the Department of Health to establish the first breast-screening unit following the publication of the Forrest report (The chairman of this commission was Professor Sir Patrick Forrest, Regius Professor of Surgery in Edinburgh, a good friend and a man I admired greatly). This unit was built near Camberwell Green in south east London and served as the training centre for the south east of England. (Figure 54) At that time I was persuaded by the

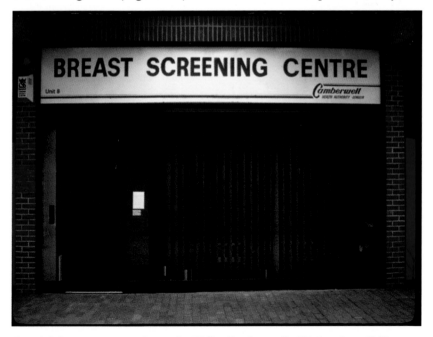

Fig. 54 Screening unit, Butterfly Walk, Camberwell, SE London, 1988

arguments in favour of screening and couldn't believe that a man of such eminence as Pat Forrest could get it wrong. As further evidence that I know a thing or two about screening, I was appointed about 8 years ago by a national agency to act as the independent chair of the national trial to evaluate prostate specific antigen (PSA) screening for the early detection of prostate cancer (ProtecT).

Suddenly in early 2009, a confluence of events threw the subject of screening for cancer into the public eye again. To start with there was the publication of a paper from the independent Nordic Cochrane Centre on mammographic screening in the BMJ in February 2009 along with an open letter to The Times signed by me amongst 27 other experts, which read as follows:

From The Times
February 19, 2009
Breast cancer screening peril
Negative consequences of the breast-screening programme

Sir,
Most people could be forgiven for believing that one of the vital weapons in the war against breast cancer is early detection even before there are any symptoms of breast cancer present. This belief has generated a Europe-wide consensus that screening healthy women for breast cancer will save lives. In the vanguard of this campaign, the NHS screening programme for breast cancer (NHS BSP) by mammography has been lauded as a triumph and has laid claim to the responsibility for the dramatic decline in breast cancer mortality since its initiation 20 years ago. An alternative view is that such success might equally well be attributed to improvements in treatment that anteceded the launch of the NHS BSP. However, there are harms associated with early detection of breast cancer by screening that are not widely acknowledged. For example, there is evidence to show that up to half of all cancers and their precursor lesions that are found by screening, if left to their own devices, might not do any harm to the woman during her natural lifespan. Yet, if found at screening, they potentially label the woman as a cancer patient: she may then be subjected to the unnecessary traumas of surgery, radiotherapy and perhaps chemotherapy, as well as suffer the potential for serious social and psychological problems. The stigma may continue to the next generation as her daughters can face higher health insurance premiums when judged as high risk. We believe that women should

*be clearly informed of these harms in order to make their own choice
about whether to attend for screening. The subject has now come to
a head with the publication in the next issue of the British Medical
Journal of "Breast screening: the facts or maybe not" by Peter C.
Gøtzsche and his colleagues from the independent Nordic Cochrane
Centre. They describe a synthesis of published papers that quantify
the benefits and harms of screening using absolute rather than
relative numbers that make it easier to comprehend. They conclude
as follows: if 2,000 women are screened regularly for ten years, one
will benefit from the screening, as she will avoid dying from breast
cancer. At the same time ten women will be treated unnecessarily.
While there is debate about exactly what these numbers are (some
data shows more women benefit and fewer healthy women treated
unnecessarily) the overall picture is clear.*

*The most disturbing statistic is that none of the invitations for
screening comes close to telling the truth. As a result, women are
being manipulated, albeit unintentionally, into attending. It is therefore
imperative that the NHS BSP rewrites the information leaflets, and leave
it to the properly informed woman to accept the invitation or not.*

*Professor Michael Baum, ChM, FRCS, MD, FRCR, FRSA
Emeritus Professor of Surgery, UCL. And 27 others*

Not long after that there were two papers published in the New
England Journal of Medicine in March, reporting on the early results
of screening for prostate cancer by using the PSA blood test. The best
case scenario that could be deduced from these data were that you
would have to screen 1,500 men for 10 years in order to save one
premature death from prostate cancer whilst at the same time treat 50
men with radical surgery for a condition that if left alone would never
threaten their life. Needless to say the overall mortality in the screened
and unscreened groups were no different from each other. For some
extraordinary reason this was accompanied by banner headlines in the
Daily Telegraph demanding PSA screening on the NHS that could
save 2,000 lives a year. Later on I will explain just how wrong this
statement was but before then it behoves me to explain some of the
delusions and illusions of screening in general.

"For every complex problem there is a simple solution – and it's
wrong"**

**Aphorism of American humorist H.L. Menken

The majority of lay people could be forgiven for believing that one of the mainstays in the fight against cancer is "early detection". This belief has generated a European-wide consensus that screening for cancer before it becomes symptomatic will save lives. It has also become the main plank in the government's campaign to improve cancer survival in the UK to match the highest levels achieved in the EU. In the vanguard of this campaign, the NHS screening programme for breast cancer (NHSBSP) by mammography has been lauded as a triumph and has laid claim to the responsibility for the dramatic decline in breast cancer mortality since its initiation more than 20 years ago. Those of us who have remained sceptical from the start have been branded as either misogynists or fools. Furthermore if it's good enough for women, what about men's health as well? How can early detection of cancer be a bad thing? Although counterintuitive, a growing body of informed opinion is moving in that direction.

Let us start by considering two separate but related issues; firstly biases of screening that give a false impression of benefit, and secondly the over-detection of cancer "look-alikes" that if left undetected might never threaten a patient's life. The survival from cancer is measured from the time of detection until recurrence and death. If a frame shift in the chronology of the disease due to screening occurs, then survival is automatically extended even if the ultimate outcome is the same; this is called lead-time bias. Of course if the "cancer" detected would never have threatened a woman's life in the first instance then that lead time might be as long as 30 years. Next, bearing in mind that the interval between screens is anything from one to three years, it is inevitable that the fast growing tumours with a bad prognosis will appear during the intervals whilst the slow growing tumours with a good prognosis will sit around until found by mammography; this is called length bias. There is also another subtle bias that can be described as the "self selection" bias. In that case women who accept invitations for screening might be demographically different to those who ignore the invitation. For a variety of reasons such women have better outcomes in the treatment of cancer forgetting whether they were screen detected or not. A recent example that goes some way to explain this bias is the fact that the same women who accept invitations for screening comply with the advice to complete 5 years of tamoxifen should they be found to have a breast cancer. Whereas the ones who don't accept the invitation and present with breast cancer don't complete their treatment. In other words the "benefit" of screening might be a surrogate marker for the success of tamoxifen.

The only way to account for these biases is to consider all the clinical trials of screening versus no screening and look for the pooled results described in terms of mortality i.e. the number of women dying in the screened group compared with those dying in the control group rather than case survival. There is in fact a modest advantage to screening looked upon in those terms, as described in the 2009 publication in the BMJ; "Breast screening: the facts – or maybe not" by Peter C Gøtzsche and his colleagues. In this milestone paper they describe a synthesis of all the papers that describe both the benefits and harms of screening using absolute rather than relative numbers that make it easy for women to comprehend, and conclude as follows…. If 2,000 women are screened regularly for 10 years, one will benefit from the screening, as she will avoid dying from breast cancer.

(The United States Preventive Services Task Force derived a similar number independently in 2004·) However even the 1:2,000 might be an over-estimate. Remember these data were derived from the trials that were mostly started in the 1970s and reported in the late 1980s. Since then improvements in treatment, such as the adoption of tamoxifen and adjuvant chemotherapy, have narrowed the window of opportunity and we have witnessed a drop in mortality of 30%–40% both in the age group that are invited for screening (>50) as well as for the younger woman. Forgetting the precise number, that one woman who benefits from a decade of screening has a life of infinite worth and if screening were as non-toxic as wearing a seat belt, there would be no case to answer. However there is a downside and that is the problem of the over-diagnosis of "pseudo-cancers". It is deduced by the Cochrane report that for every life saved 10 healthy women will, as a consequence, become cancer patients and will be treated unnecessarily. These women will have either a part of their breast or the whole breast removed, and they will often receive radiotherapy and sometimes chemotherapy. This is the tricky part of the story that is more or less denied by the screening fraternity and therefore deserves some close attention.

Screening for breast cancer is now adopted as an unequivocal good by most of the members of the EU. Invitations for screening promote this activity by being economical with the truth. One of the uncomfortable truths concerns the over-diagnosis of both in-situ and invasive breast cancers in screening populations. Over-diagnosis of breast cancer doesn't mean false positive rates. It means the detection and treatment of cancers that left undetected would never threaten a woman's life and with which she would live, in blissful unawareness, until she died naturally of old age. We had always assumed that there was an over-diagnosis of duct carcinoma in-situ (DCIS), some of which had the potential of progressing to an invasive and life-threatening phenotype. However, there is now clear evidence that anything between 10% and 50% of invasive cancers detected and treated radically as a result of screening, would never threaten life. As a result the overall mastectomy rate *rises* after any country implements screening in contrast to the message in the NHSBSP leaflet, "*breast cancer the facts*" that implies that screening saves breasts. It doesn't.

How can this possibly be? Don't we know that if cancer is neglected it will progress to a life-threatening condition?

By way of illumination let me propose that the pathological diagnosis of cancer at screening is based on a *syllogism;* (a *syllogism* is a logical argument in three propositions, two premises and a conclusion, the conclusion being specious) A simple example might be the fact that Van Gogh was a genius of an artist who never sold a painting in his lifetime, I am an artist who has never sold a painting *ergo*: I'm an unrecognized genius. Another example from the practice of medicine goes like this; people who die from meningitis harbour meningococci in their nose. This does not mean that harbouring meningococci in the nose is a lethal condition; in fact about 10% of the population harbour these bacteria.

Cancer was defined by its microscopic appearance about two hundred years ago. The 19th century saw the birth of scientific oncology with the discovery and use of the modern microscope. Rudolf Virchow, often called the founder of cellular pathology, provided the scientific basis for the modern pathologic study of cancer. As earlier generations had correlated the autopsy findings observed with the unaided eye with the clinical course of cancer one hundred years earlier, so Virchow correlated the microscopic pathology of the disease.

However the material he was studying came from the autopsy of patients *dying* from cancer. In the mid 19thC pathological correlations were performed on living subjects presenting with locally advanced or metastatic disease that almost always were pre-determined to die in the absence of effective therapy. Since then, without pause for thought, the microscopic identification of cancer according to these classic criteria has been associated with the assumed prognosis of a fatal disease if left untreated. The syllogism at the heart of the diagnosis of cancer therefore runs like this; people frequently die from malignant disease, under the microscope this malignant disease has many histological features we will call "cancer", *ergo:* anything that looks like "cancer" under the microscope will kill you. I would therefore like to argue that some of these earliest stages of "cancer", if left unperturbed, would not progress to a disease with lethal potential. These "pseudo-cancers" might have microscopic similarity to true cancers but these appearances are only a necessary rather than sufficient condition for a fatal disease. I would also like to suggest that many of the "risk factors" for the development of cancer are in fact the promotional agents of a latent condition that Gilbert Welch has described as pseudo-cancers.

If we stand back to take a broader look at nature this shouldn't be surprising. Conventional mathematical models of cancer growth are linear or logarithmic, in other words completely predictable at the outset. These mathematical formulae may be appropriate for designing theme park rides but cannot begin to explain the exquisite organization of cell proliferation and the complex inter-relationships of cells of different progeny.

Most natural biological mechanisms are non-linear or better described according to chaos theory. The beauty of the tree in full leaf reflects its fractal geometry that looks remarkably similar to the microscopic appearance of the mammary ducts and lobules under the microscope. The rate of growth and the development of the lung along with the fingers and toes in the foetus cannot be described in linear terms. Another example might be wound healing that starts with the surgeon's knife and ends with a perfect scar that should be almost invisible, although rarely wound healing carries on too long to leave an ugly keloid scar. Prolonged latency followed by catastrophe should not be all that surprising. We accept the case for prostate cancer, as we know that most elderly men will die *with* prostate cancer in situ and not *of* prostate cancer that has invaded. In fact the UK national PSA screening trial is predicated on that fact with two a priori outcome measures defined, deaths from prostate cancer versus the number of cancers treated unnecessarily. Why oh why does the breast cancer lobby remain in denial? Of course now that the cat is out of the bag they will have no choice but to include this fact in their invitations in order to avoid litigation from an irate woman in the future. Furthermore "the sins of the mother are visited on the daughter". We now have cases of women with screen-detected DCIS whose daughters have had problems raising mortgages when the insurers have discovered this family history of breast cancer!

By way of a minor diversion I want briefly to discuss prostate cancer screening. In my preamble I mentioned the banner headlines in one of our respected broadsheets following the publications in the New England Journal of Medicine in March 2009. Unlike the writers of that piece I actually read the publications and not just the press release of a prostate cancer charity. There were in fact two studies reported together with a lengthy editorial. The first study was American and produced a negative result. The larger European study was of borderline statistical significance and for the statistically literate amongst you, showed a 20% relative risk reduction of cancer specific mortality over a 10 year period with a p value of <0.04. Never mind the stats, translated into numbers that all laymen could understand, you would need to screen about 1,500 men for 10 years to save one prostate cancer death at the expense of over-diagnosing close to 50 cases of cancer that would be treated with radical surgery that frequently leads to impotence and incontinence and on rare occasions death from the complications of surgery. The editorial concluded that it was premature to make any kind of recommendation and urged that we waited for the outcome of the British trial. That happens to be the study I chair. I can claim no credit for the elegant and ambitious design of that trial that is all down to the three principal investigators, Freddie Hamdy, Jenny Donovan and David Neal. I was invited in as an independent chairman to see fair play. 500,000 men in the UK have been randomized to PSA screening or not. Those with a raised PSA are further investigated and if in the end their prostate biopsies showed localized cancer they are then offered re-randomization to three treatment groups, radical surgery, radical radiotherapy or "active monitoring". The two primary outcome measures are cancer specific mortality and the rate of over-diagnosis. Health economics is factored in as well and the secondary randomization will allow measures of quality of life as well as length of life in the different treatment groups, whilst the "active monitoring" arm will allow us to study the natural history of screen-detected prostate cancer. This latter group will also allow us to study the molecular biology of the disease to see if we can learn to separate out the "poodles" (cancers that will remain latent for the duration of life) from the "Rottweilers" (those that are predetermined to invade and spread). If only we had our time over again *that* is how the breast cancer trials should have been designed!

So is there a reasonable "exit strategy" that will save face and serve womankind the better? Let me summarize in a series of bullet points where we have arrived with breast cancer screening.

- The current NHS screening programme is based on the results of randomized controlled trials that were published before 1987 and started in the late 1960s and early 1970s

- Some of these trials in retrospect were of poor quality

- With mature follow up and careful attention to biases, a relative risk reduction (RRR) in breast cancer specific mortality has been estimated as 15%

- In absolute terms therefore the numbers needed to screen over 10 years to prevent one breast cancer death is about 1:2,000. Anything better than this depends on ignoring the obvious biases in the trials, mathematical manipulation of the data that I either simply don't understand or is based on those self-selected women who accept the invitation to screen. ("Selection bias")

- Along the way the estimates of harm have increased. At the outset the hazards of over-diagnosis were ignored, then as the rate of screen detected duct carcinoma in situ (DCIS) shot up it was still judged to be worth the cost. Now we recognize that the over-diagnosis of invasive cancers (IDC), that are not predestined to threaten a woman's life, is a problem. The extent of over-diagnosis is debatable but I personally agree that if you include DCIS and IDC it mounts to about 10 cases treated unnecessarily for every life saved.

- Putting politics aside for the moment I wonder how many of us would have voted for the NHSBSP in 1987 knowing what we know today.

- Furthermore in spite of the wonderful advances we've made in imaging technology and treatment in the last 20 years there has been only one new trial reported for screening and that was the trial for the under 50s that supported the 15% estimate.

- In other words we are using state of the art imaging and modern therapy to service a programme based on data that is 20 years old.

It is also worth re-iterating at this juncture that improvements in the treatment of symptomatic patients since the mid 1980s leaves a much narrower window of opportunity for screening so that even our estimates of 1: 2,000 based on these old trials might have to be adjusted.

So where do we go from here? To close the programme is politically unacceptable. I therefore want to make two practical propositions for research and development. One concerns "person preferences" and the other concerns the more efficient use of scarce resources that I will refer to as risk assessment/risk management (RARM)

Since 1997 when I resigned from the NHSBS committee in disgust about the way women were being coerced into screening, I have publicly expressed my concerns on the issue of informed choice. This has often led to ridicule and *ad hominem* attacks.

I take no particular pleasure in the fact that the NHS has at last accepted the point and agreed to rewrite the letters of invitation.

From The Times February 21, 2009
"NHS rips up breast cancer leaflet and starts all over again"

My concern is that they will repeat the mistakes of the past if we leave this task to the usual suspects. Furthermore it's not for me to prejudge what level of benefit and what level of harm might influence the average woman to accept the invitation. For this reason I think there are two related areas of research. First the development of an information pack that includes decision aids. This could be used in a person preference study where well women might be offered sliding scales of benefits and harms to find the point at which screening is judged acceptable. These data might then inform the next and perhaps more important area of research on more efficient ways of using scarce resources in the NHS.

The beauty of a risk assessment risk management is that it provides a platform for the management of all women in an attempt to reduce the mortality from breast cancer where mammographic screening is one component of an integrated programme. The first step is to set up a facility nationwide for risk assessment using one of the modern computer programmes. Women would then be *offered* not *compelled* to accept this service. Initially a practice nurse could administer this questionnaire but it would be quite easy to transfer this to a web-based programme for the computer literate members of the community. From the read-out an initial triage could be agreed. Those at the most extreme end of the risk spectrum, say with a relative risk (RR) of say >10.0, could be invited to a clinical genetics consultation. At the other extreme those with a RR of say <2.0 might be reassured and given lifestyle advice on diet, alcohol and exercise. (Please note that these risk ratios are for illustration only, the actual figures used could be derived from the person preference studies and the cut-off for genetic counselling is already broadly accepted) Those in between could then be invited to a special clinic for the second step. At this clinic women of 45 or older could have a mammogram to determine breast density that might also be kept as a baseline but also provide additional evidence about risk. (The greater the mammographic density the higher the risk) Those with radiological abnormality at this stage would be investigated in the accepted way. If the mammographic density is low and the repeat estimate falls below a RR of 2.0 then they would be reassured and given lifestyle advice. Incidentally lifestyle advice concerning exercise, weight control, diet, alcohol and tobacco as well as reducing the risk of dying from cancer will incidentally reduce the risk of premature death from stroke or heart disease that is at least 25 times more likely than death from breast cancer.

To carry on regardless is no longer acceptable, neither is political spin the answer. Women are now getting smarter and the demand for change doesn't just come from grumpy old men like me but also from the legions of wise women represented by the signatories of the letter in The Times. However the changes I have in mind are not destructive but constructive. The NHSBSP has indirectly lead to the provision of the best specialist services for the diagnosis and treatment of symptomatic breast cancer in the world, riding on the back of the screening units.

It is the centralization of care leading to the rapid recruitment into RCTs for the treatment of cancer that is the major contributor to the dramatic fall in breast cancer mortality in the UK over the last two decades. If we can now add to this the prevention of stroke, heart disease and lung cancer with a risk adjusted screening programme then everyone will be a winner.

Chapter 17

The Prince and the Pauper

In February 2008 I was asked by the BMJ to respond to Prince Charles' advocacy of alternative medicine. I did so by way of an open letter that I reproduce below in full.

'With respect your Highness you've got it wrong'.

Your Royal Highness,

20 years ago, on the occasion of the 150th anniversary of the British Medical Association (BMA), you were appointed our President and used your position to admonish my profession for its complacency. You also took advantage of this platform to promote "alternative" medicine. Shortly after that I enjoyed the privilege of meeting with you at a series of colloquia organized by the Royal Society of Medicine (RSM) to debate the role of complementary and alternative medicine (CAM) in health care.

Of course you won't remember me but the event is indelible in my memory. I was the only one amongst my professional colleagues to unequivocally register dissent. At the cocktail party to mark the closure of our meetings I had the impertinence to say that although I disagreed with you about "alternative" medicine you were absolutely right about the architects. (I'm sure you remember the "carbuncle" episode). Quick as a flash you described how the previous night, having dinner at the Royal Institute of British Architects (RIBA), you were accosted by a prominent architect who stated that you were absolutely wrong about British architecture but he couldn't agree more about your stand on British Medicine! From that point onwards you won my undying devotion.

A few days later you were rewarded with a four-page supplement in the London Evening Standard, promoting unproven cures for cancer and I was invited by the same journal to respond. I requested the same space but was only allowed one page, which at the last minute was cut by a quarter to make space for an advert for a new release by "Frankie Goes to Hollywood". Furthermore the sub-editors embarrassed me with the banner headline, "With respect your Highness, you've got it wrong". (The Standard August 13th 1984). As I have nothing more to lose I'm happy for that headline to grace the BMJ today.

Over the last 20 years I have treated thousands of patients with cancer and lost some dear friends and relatives along the way with this dreaded disease. I guess that for the majority of my patients their first meeting with me was as momentous and memorable as mine was with you. Sadly, however hard I try, many of these courageous men and women are not instantly recognized and covertly I check their notes before each follow up in order to practice the benign deception of greeting them like long lost friends. This phenomenon of asymmetrical relationships I like to describe as the "gradient of power". The power of my authority comes with a knowledge built on 40 years of study and 25 years of active involvement in cancer research. I'm sensitive to the danger of abusing this power and as a last resort I know that the General Medical Council (GMC) is watching over my shoulder to ensure I respect a code of conduct with a duty of care that respects a patient's dignity and privacy and reminds me that my personal beliefs should not prejudice my advice.

If you will forgive me sir, your power and authority rests on an accident of birth. Furthermore, as illustrated above, your public utterances are worthy of four pages, whereas if lucky I might warrant one. I don't begrudge you that authority and we probably share many opinions about Art and Architecture, but I do beg of you to exercise your power with extreme caution when advising patients with life threatening diseases to embrace unproven therapies. There is no equivalent of the GMC for the monarchy, so it is left to either sensational journalists or more rarely the quiet voice of loyal subjects such as myself, to warn you that you may have overstepped the mark. It is in the nature of your world to be surrounded by sycophants (including members of the medical establishment hungry for their mention in the Queen's birthday honours' list) who constantly reinforce what they assume are your prejudices. Last week I had a sense of déja-vu, when you welcomed the BMA representatives to Llandudno for the annual meeting and later appeared in The Observer (June 27th) and Daily Express (June 28th) promoting coffee enemas and carrot juice for cancer. Much has changed since you shocked us out of our complacency 20+ years ago.

The GMC is reformed and as part of this revolution so has our undergraduate teaching. Professional development is part of our student's core curriculum, involving modules in the Humanities. Students are taught the importance of the spiritual domain but at the same time study the epistemology of Medicine, or in simpler words the nature of proof. Many lay people have an impressionistic notion of science as a cloak for bigotry. Nothing could be further from the truth. The scientific method is based on the deductive process that starts with the humble assumption that your hypothesis might be wrong and is then subjected to experiments that carry the risk of falsification. This approach works. For example in my own specialist disease, breast cancer, we have witnessed a 30% fall in mortality since 1984, resulting from a worldwide collaboration in clinical trials, accompanied by improvements in quality of life as measured by psychometric instruments. You promote the Gerson diet whose only support comes from inductive logic i.e. anecdote. I have Gerson's book on my desk as I write. Forget the implausible rationale, simply search for anything other than testimonial support. What is wrong with anecdote you may ask? After all these are real human-interest stories. The problems are manifold but start with the assumption that cancer has a predictable natural history. "The patient was only given 6 months to live, tried the diet and lived for years". This is an urban myth. None of us are so arrogant as to predict that which is known only to the Almighty. With advanced breast cancer the median expectation of life might be 18 months, but many of my patients live for many years longer, with or without treatment. I have always advocated the scientific evaluation of CAM using controlled trials and **if** *"alternative" therapies pass these rigorous tests of so called "orthodox" medicine, then they will cease to be alternative and join our armamentarium. If their proponents lack the courage of their convictions to have their pet remedies subjected to the "hazards of refutation" then they are the bigots who will forever be condemned to practise on the fringe.*

I have much time for complimentary therapy that offers improvements in quality of life or spiritual solace, providing that it is truly integrated with modern medicine, but I have no time at all for "alternative" therapy which places itself above the laws of evidence and practices in a metaphysical domain that harks back to the dark days of Galen.

The "post-modern" philosophers, with their talk of post-Enlightenment hegemony, would have us believe that all knowledge is relative and the dominance of one belief system is determined by the power of its proponents. The hazards of this way of thinking are beautifully exposed in Francis Wheen's new book, "How Mumbo-Jumbo Conquered the World". Instead, perhaps we should all remain cognizant of the words of the Nobel Lauriat, Jacques Monod; "Personal self-satisfaction is the death of the scientist. Collective self-satisfaction is the death of the research. It is restlessness, anxiety, dissatisfaction, agony of mind that nourish science". Please your Royal Highness; help us nourish medical science by sharing our agony.

Yours Sincerely,
Michael Baum

As you can imagine the ceiling fell in on me after that was published, I rapidly found out who my true friends were and I was jokingly told that I could kiss my knighthood good bye. In my defence I can claim that I've studied complimentary and alternative medicine (CAM) for a long while and written many papers on the subject. Furthermore I have chaired two European committees on the role of CAM in cancer and for three years chaired the psychosocial oncology committee of our National Cancer Research Network (NCRN). I now want to describe my thoughts on the subject in detail.

Patients diagnosed with cancer have many needs. The diagnosis comes as a shock and maybe for the first time, the individual is facing up to her mortality. So before health service providers even think about the role of medicine, they must consider patients' needs for moral and spiritual support. At times like this, a close supportive family and membership of a faith community are invaluable. Sadly there are many cancer sufferers who lack family support and have no spiritual mentor. Perhaps one explanation of the growth in the interest in CAM is the unmet need of the patient when conventional medical practice fails to fill this aching void.

The next need for cancer subjects is to be free of whatever symptoms plague their life, as a result of the disease. Of course, in the early stages the patients may be symptom free but, in the later stages, suffering is common from pain, nausea and weakness. The science of pain control is well established and palliative care for those close to the end is a well-developed specialty thanks to the British hospice movement. In addition there may well be a role for interventions such as therapeutic massage and counselling to help the patient feel better. Relatively new is the discipline of "Psycho-social oncology" which aims to identify and manage the more subtle subjective symptoms of cancer such as anxiety and depression. This field of activity emerged about 20 years ago with the development of psychometric instruments. It addresses the psychological, social, spiritual and behavioural dimensions of being afflicted with the diagnosis of cancer from both perspectives: the one of the patient and the ones of the members of his or her social network. Furthermore there exists a mind/body nexus that, in theory, could be modulated to influence the natural course of the disease so that if the patient "feels better" it might indirectly help them "get better".

The third need of cancer victims is to be cured or at least have their lives prolonged. I have described in detail in earlier chapters of this book how we have set about achieving this goal.

We still have a long way to go and once again there is no room for complacency. The challenge for the oncologists of today is to get the correct balance between the curiosity (scientific interest in helping patients of the future) and the compassion (helping patients of the present) in order to reach the optimal efficiency level of care both in routine clinical practice and for the patient treated in the context of clinical research. Against this background let us consider the meaning of complementary and alternative medicine (CAM).

The English language has a rich and beautiful vocabulary. All these wonderful words have precise meaning and we tamper with them at our peril. George Orwell's terrifying book 1984 illustrates the ultimate triumph of the evil of a totalitarian state. By the simple device of distorting the language as to make it impossible to even harbour subversive thoughts, "Big Brother" ruled absolutely. It saddens me to witness how the language is being debased by a pseudo-culture that encourages transient values and transient meanings to our vocabulary. The same worry concerns the use of the words "alternative" and "complementary" when applied to the practice of medicine.

The first question you have to ask about "alternative" is – alternative to what? Proponents of alternative medicine will describe the practice of doctors in the National Health Service, both in primary and tertiary care, as "orthodox", "mainstream", "Western", "reductionist", and so on. In return the practitioners of conventional medicine view "alternative/unconventional" medicine as a series of comprehensive health belief systems, superficially with little in common, yet sharing beliefs in metaphysical concepts of balance and similarities which date back to Galenic doctrine from the second century A.D, or oriental mysticism 2,000 years older. So in this parallel universe of alternative medicine, treatments are based on metaphysical concepts, rather than orthodox physiology and biochemistry. Yet it has to be accepted that each view of the other is to some extent pejorative, and if we are to establish a dialogue between the champions on either side of this conceptual divide we must show mutual trust and mutual respect. Perhaps for the time being we might blur these distinctions by using the word "unproven" which can apply equally well to therapeutic interventions on each side. Of course, the issue of the definition of "proof" then raises problems that I will address later.

Next we must consider the definition of "complementary". The Oxford English Dictionary defines the word as, "that which completes or makes perfect, or that which when added completes a whole." In other words, whilst modern medical science struggles to cure patients, complementary medicine helps patients to feel better, and who knows, by feeling better the act of healing itself may be complemented. Some complementary approaches may be placebos, and the touch of the "healer" or the hand of the massage therapist could be guided by strange belief systems that are alien to modern science. Providing the intention is to support the clinician in his endeavours rather than compete in the relativistic market place of ideas one might set aside these concerns.

The prevalence of CAM usage in the world can no longer be ignored by the practitioners of evidence-based medicine. This is relevant to medical practice in a number of ways. First of all it must reflect the unmet needs of cancer patients. Secondly we have a duty of care to protect our patients from the dangers of remedies that might be toxic, interact unfavourably with our own medications or be promoted as alternatives to evidence based treatment.

The massive emotional impact after the disclosure of diagnosis of cancer can result in fear, confusion and isolation. The fear can be countered by reassurance and the offer of hope by the responsible clinician. Hope is not a promise but a state of mind. Confusion can be countered by improvement in the communication skills of the practitioner. I welcome the developments in the undergraduate and

197

post-graduate curricula designed to teach professional development and communication skills. At the same time the negative judgment on the medical profession made by some CAM practitioners and representatives of the media regarding the concern about the subjective outcomes of medical care must be challenged. It should be remembered that surgical and medical oncologists were the first to invent, critically evaluate and implement quality of life measurement tools. In addition, counselling is well accepted by the nursing and the medical profession. Here for a start is a non-controversial way of building bridges among all professionals involved.

Beyond that, the popularity of CAM might reflect the time constraints of medical practitioners in understaffed and underfunded government health services, unrealistic expectations of the patient for the best that modern medicine can offer, a desperation of the patient or her family in facing up to the terminal stages of the disease, or even a cultural/philosophical objection to modern medicine which is one component of the post modern relativistic philosophy popular in parts of Europe today.

All "believers" and "non-believers" accept that there is a transcendental component to life that can offer comfort, support and an explanation for the "human condition". Atheists might gain this through fine art, music, literature, poetry and theatre. "Believers", in addition to their access to the arts, may achieve the transcendental via membership of a faith community or by seeking their spiritual salvation through any number of "new-age" belief systems. However spiritual comfort is achieved, focusing on the transcendental enhances a sense of personal control, builds self esteem, offers a meaning to both life and death, provides comfort and hope, and if "believers" are members of an organized faith community, they will have access to community support. Of course belief in God and belief in modern medicine are not mutually exclusive. However, there can be a down side to all this, if religiosity is confused with magic or subverted to be in conflict with a doctor's duty of care.

Even the word "healing" is open to semantic abuse using the term in a loose way to imply "healing of the spirit" rather than the common usage where "to heal" is meant "to cure". Some charlatans appear content to allow this misconception to stand uncorrected yet deny ever claiming that their interventions contributed to a cure. Others, who truly believe in their healing powers as a cure, often invoke a view of a lost "golden age" when nature offered a cure for all human ailments. In this respect medical practitioners must take a robust position. There never was such a "golden age", nature is neutral and "left to nature" would mean observing the natural history of cancer. At the same time "golden age" beliefs imply a denial of progress. Most sinister of all are the faith systems that look upon disease as "God's will" and cancer as some kind of punishment, in which case "healing" can only follow prayer. This is an evil doctrine equivalent to those who claimed that the victims of the tsunami disaster reflected God's anger at mankind's corruption.

In order to promote a dialogue and for the sake of our patients, it would be helpful to lay to rest the myth that doctors working in the conventional health care systems are knowingly denying patients the proven benefits of therapeutic strategies developed by proponents of CAM. If there is evidence for the claims linked to an intervention, then it doesn't matter what their point of origin or provenance might be. In return, if approached by professionals engaged in CAM for help in testing whether their favoured intervention is of value, then it should be the responsibility of the medical establishment to assist the best they can. What has to be agreed, however, is there cannot be a double standard. In the broadest terms there are three categories of research design involving cancer patients.

Firstly there is "qualitative research" which usually has the intention of capturing the individual patient's experience and defining their needs. This in itself does not provide evidence of efficacy of an individual treatment but should be used to set the agenda for other research models. Next there is observational research that is the tool of epidemiologists. They might provide clues to suggest therapies e.g. dietary intervention, or more importantly on the prevention of disease. Finally there is the clinical trial. It is at this point we have to consider the randomised controlled trial (RCT). This study design is sufficiently robust to cope with the extraordinary variability and to some extent unpredictability of cancer. The properly designed and conducted RCT therefore can control for case mix, selection bias, observer bias and placebo effect and is sufficiently malleable to accommodate the needs of CAM. For example if the CAM intervention is aimed at improving quality of life (QOL) or patient satisfaction then these can be defined as primary endpoints and measured by one or more of the many psychometric instruments that have already been validated. If the primary endpoint is not already covered by one of the instruments, for example in the spiritual domain, then the onus should be on its proponent to develop a new instrument; remembering Lord Kalvin's aphorism "if it exists then you can measure it". Another problem that has to be accommodated concerns the individualization of treatment often used as an excuse to avoid RCTs. Here again a robust design would allow randomisation of the "individualized" intervention against a non-individualized "one size fits all" treatment, and let the best man win.

Clinical trials often generate results that are not entirely in agreement with each other. Thus it is misleading to rely on the finding one prefers and to omit those one doesn't like. In other words, we have to consider the totality of the available data. Systematic reviews (SR) are attempts to summarize and evaluate the totality of the available evidence of a pre-defined nature on a certain subject. All the components of the approach and assessment are made explicit so that the result is entirely reproducible. If statistical pooling is used, this is called a meta-analysis. The strength of systematic reviews is that they minimize selection (i.e. the emphasis on the trials that reinforce a prejudice) and the play of chance. Thus they can provide the most objective evidence on a given subject and are a sound basis for clinical decisions. The same standards of quality must be used for CAM and for mainstream medicine. A double standard situation is not acceptable.

I believe that, should a promising treatment one day emerge from "alternative" therapy, it should be investigated without delay by oncologists and adopted into routine care as soon as the data supporting its use are sufficiently strong. For example plant-based cancer medications such as Vincristin and Vinblastin (both using extract from the plant *Vinca rosea*) or Taxol (*Taxus baccata*) are already in routine use.

Although I have often been outspoken in my criticism of proponents of CAM, one thing we must all accept is that practitioners of conventional medicine and practitioners of CAM are working in good faith to improve the length and quality of life for patients with cancer. The way forward is to build bridges, but I predict these bridges will never be completed because of the subversion by the increasingly vocal anti-science lobby in the UK.

It is at this point I would like to have a sideswipe at homeopathy – my personal bête noire.

On September 1st 2006, The Medicines for Human Use (National rules for Homeopathic Products) Regulations Statutory Instrument 2006 No. 1952 came into force. As a headline that has an impact factor a little below "Small earthquake in Peru, few killed". Yet by my reasoning this might be an early symptom of a malaise that is polluting our culture. The Medicines for Human Use Regulatory Agency (MHRA) came into being following the Medicines Act in 1968 to provide strict rules for licensing new medicines based on evidence of safety and efficacy following the thalidomide tragedy. All medicinal products on the market at that time were granted automatic product licences with the view of revisiting them in due course for evidence of safety and efficacy, but all new products had to pass these stringent rules. When Britain joined the European Common Market in 1973, evidence of safety and efficacy for all medicines became mandatory *except for homeopathy*, which enjoyed a privileged place. New homeopathic remedies could not be marketed as they couldn't provide efficacy data that would be required of conventional medicines. EC directive 2001/83 provided member states the opportunity to manage this discrepancy in the licensing of conventional and orthodox medicines. Sweden for example elected for a single standard of evidence, as a result of which new homeopathic remedies will never become available in that eminently rational country. By contrast, the UK Statutory instrument 2006 No. 1952 demonstrated that Britain no longer rules the waves but as far as homeopathy is concerned, waives the rules, introducing a double standard of breathtaking *chutzpah*.*

As always the devil is in the detail and clouded in officialese. *Viz.* Section 1 subsection 1(a)

- "An application for the grant of a UK marketing authorization for a national homeopathic product is **not** (my emphasis) required to be made in accordance with -(a) the second and third indents of Article 8.3(i) of the 2001 Directive, the requirement to submit results of pre-clinical and clinical trials".

There again in Part 3 Evidence of efficacy, section 6 (c);

- "The data must consist of at least the results of investigations, commonly known as homeopathic "provings", which consist of the administration of a substance to a human subject in order to ascertain the symptoms produced by that substance."

Translated into English what that means is that homeopathy is spared from submitting the results of randomized controlled trials (RCTs)

---

*Chutzpah; A Yiddish word whose nearest English equivalent might be "bloody cheek".

for evidence of efficacy but instead it would be acceptable to offer evidence obtained from "provings". Equal weight is therefore given to the evidence of scientific trials for modern medicines and *"Similia similibus curentur"* (the magic of similarities) for homeopathy.

Friday September 1st dawned with yet another morning of surrealistic debate over the airwaves followed by an afternoon and evening where art imitated life. I turned up at 7.00 am in the studios of the Today programme with a sense of *déjà vu* all over again, to be cross-examined by the presenter John Humphries and to be joined by the out-of-body voice of Dr. Fisher, spokesman for the Royal London Homeopathic Hospital (RLHH). There was nothing paranormal about his presence. It was just another example of the miracle of modern science whereby he could join us on air via electromagnetic waves transmitted from his cell phone in the wilds of Scotland, via some passing orbiting satellite to the studio and then out from there to the world at large. The most extraordinary comment from Dr. Fisher was an expression of satisfaction that at last homeopathy and orthodox medicine would be enjoying a level playing field! Eh?! I watched Arsenal draw with Middleborough one all, the previous Saturday, in their beautiful new Emirates Stadium. The playing field looked as level as a snooker table and at my count there were 11 men a side (although to be fair one of the 'Borough's defenders was sent off for the last 10 minutes of the game). How is it a level playing field for the pharmaceutical Industry to have to submit the results of RCTs with thousands of patients, years of follow up, Good Clinical Practice (GCP) standards of governance and careful statistical analysis for efficacy and safety, followed by a year or two of delay awaiting reports of cost-effectiveness from National Institute of Clinical Excellence (NICE); when all the homeopathy industry has to offer is the evidence that a substance, that is retained in the "memory of water" *(vide infra)*, can induce symptoms of a disease, if given in its natural state?

My next interview was on BBC breakfast television in the company of a charming young lady representing the society of homeopaths. She was brandishing a bottle of Arnica 30C, which she assured the viewing millions was a proven remedy for bruising and minor trauma. Arnica is an extract of a yellow flower, *arnica Montana* and 30C means that it has been diluted in a volume larger than the Pacific Ocean. Water would have to have a very remarkable and selective memory in order to recall that it had once been in contact with arnica at this level of dilution! Although there is no plausible reason why it should work my companion assured the audience that there was proof of its efficacy. Apart from the fact that all systematic reviews of RCTs have failed to show that any homeopathic remedy was anything other than a placebo, I happened to know of a trial of Arnica 30C carried out by the Blackie Foundation of the RLHH, for perineal trauma after traumatic births, which was negative. I sat on their advisory board at the time and insisted that the trial should be published but it never was. When I challenged the young lady about this publication bias she was quick to boast that many negative trials (!!!) for Arnica 30C had been published, without realizing the contradiction she had just made.

As chance would have it, I was meeting Professor Donald Marcus from Baylor University for lunch that day, after which I took him to the National Gallery for a "ward round". He shares my interest in the teaching of medical humanities and I wanted to show him some of the paintings that I use to instruct medical students. Amongst the English 18C works we both admire is a delightful series by Hogarth, entitled "Marriage a la Mode". The last frame in this narrative shows the dying syphilitic wayward wife with her crippled syphilitic daughter clutching the hem of her dress. (Most of the characters in this morality play seem to be suffering from sexually transmitted diseases). On one side of this picture we can witness the servant and the apothecary indulging in a bout of fisticuffs. Hogarth completed this work in about 1742 when there was little to choose for lack of efficacy between the nostrums of the quacks and the potions of the apothecary. Dr. Samuel Hahnemann "discovered" homeopathy about 50 years later and its initial success can be ascribed to the fact that the nothingness of homeopathy must have been preferable to the bleeding, cupping, leeches, purgation, laudanum and quicksilver provided by the university educated doctors of that period; In other words the placebo effect of the doctor's gravitas minus the toxic effects of his pharmacopoeia.

The following evening my wife and I attended a charity performance of Donizetti's "L'Elisir d'Amore". Donizetti was born in northern Italy round about the time homeopathy was invented. In this comic opera (The Elixir of Love) an itinerant quack sells a potion that promises to make men irresistible to women. A local yokel is so convinced by its power that the placebo effect gives him the confidence to win back his long lost love. Donizetti sends up the placebo effects of quack remedies and the gullibility of a naïve public with delightful music and song. This work is as relevant now as it was when first performed. (Donizetti himself died a horrible, protracted death from syphilis, against which contemporary medicine was impotent.)

I have been accused by many of my good friends of wasting my time by "tilting at windmills" and will never win the argument. Maybe so – but I happen to believe that what we are witnessing is a very dangerous trend. I'm not out to win but only to fight the good fight. I think it both dangerous at a clinical level but even more so at a broader social level.

Most sceptics look upon homeopathy as a harmless placebo. Indeed that might be the case but the dangers of homeopathy are indirect. First, if a doctor prescribes it knowingly as a placebo, then he is guilty of deceit. There may be a case for such interventions for children but if used in adults it stinks of paternalism. Furthermore when a kindly doctor offers evidence-based medicine the placebo effect comes with it unintentionally, as an add-on, for free.

Next, if homeopathy is licensed for the treatment of specific symptoms then that might encourage the patient to delay seeing the doctor and serious conditions might be overlooked.

Finally, the homeopathic remedies might be seen as an alternative to a proven treatment and individuals might be putting their life at risk. A recent example was seen in the BBC Newsnight production that showed that many pharmacies are marketing homeopathic anti-malarial preparations. This seems to have coincided with the experience of the London School of Hygiene and Tropical Medicine's experience with young back-packers coming back from sub-Saharan Africa with acute malaria.

I agree with my friendly critics, who even include my wife of 40 years, that I cannot win the argument. I can think of four explanations for my pessimism and they don't make edifying reading.

First there is the danger from within. I've noted an increasing tendency amongst young general practitioners to embrace the teachings of homeopathy. They have come to believe that this marks them out as modern, caring and open minded. How is it modern to embrace a belief system that is over 200 years old? Maybe in this topsy-turvy *Erewhon* world of ours it would be even more modern to embrace Galenic teachings again, as they are 1800 years old. (Incidentally the Gerson diet favoured as alternative therapy for cancer **is** neo-Galenism). How is it caring to offer placebos with deceitful intent? How is it open minded to accept a closed dogmatic belief that has conspicuously failed to describe any breakthroughs since its invention?

The problem here is the medical profession itself is losing confidence in the scientific method and beginning to believe all the anti-science rhetoric of the tabloid media.

The next reason for my pessimism is the scientific illiteracy of the lay public that hasn't moved much since CP Snow spelt it out in his Rede Lecture (1959) "The two cultures and the Scientific Revolution".

"Closing the gap between our cultures is a necessity in the most abstract intellectual sense, as well as in the most practical. When those two senses have grown apart, then no society is going to be able to think with wisdom. For the sake of the intellectual life, for the sake of this country's special danger, for the sake of this Western society living precariously rich among the poor, for the sake of the poor who needn't be poor if there is intelligence in the world, it is obligatory for us to look at our education with fresh eyes."

Nearly 50 years later, if anything things have got worse. Fewer and fewer of our sixth formers are studying the sciences because they are considered as too difficult and irrelevant. More and more are taking "soft options" such as sociology and media studies. Departments of chemistry and physics are now closing down in our universities. Yet there is no expression of shame. Instead young people may take pride in their scientific illiteracy, blaming science for all the ills in the world and accusing science of spoiling this green and pleasant land. I'm not alone in thinking this. Lord Bragg, that great writer, broadcaster and polymath, described these phenomena in his book "On Giants' Shoulders: Great Scientists and Their Discoveries, from Archimedes to DNA", as did Lord Taverne in his book "The March of Unreason", and neither is a scientist.

This latter book also introduces my next concern and that is the growing power of post-modern relativism. The creeping success of this French school of philosophy with its impenetrable use of language has replaced the need for critical thought on our campuses. As all systems of belief are equally valid, culturally determined and value laden, then anything goes. It is now considered extremely bad form if I suggest I know more about breast cancer than a patient suffering from the disease. Furthermore, as it is a well known fact that there is a conspiracy of the Government, the medical establishment and the pharmaceutical industry to risk the health of young children with immunization regimens, then it is perfectly reasonable for the modern and caring "yummy mummy" to avoid this threat and protect their children with natural remedies. To argue otherwise is an expression of heuristic, triumphalistic, Western industrial bio-scientific global hegemony (or words to that effect).

My final concern relates to the opinion that belief in the irrational and supernatural is "hard wired" (genetically predetermined). This was a topic of debate at the British Association for Advancement of Science at the University of East Anglia in September 2007. In a brilliant lecture, Professor Bruce Hood from the University of Bristol described an extraordinary series of experiments to demonstrate that scientists' efforts to combat "irrational" beliefs are ultimately futile. For example even the most sceptical scientists would not swap their wedding rings for identical replicas. Attaching sentimental significance to inanimate objects is little different to belief in the supernatural. He argued that this capacity of the human mind to think intuitively and to develop theories had some evolutionary advantages. I disagree. Professor Lewis Wolpert of University College London (he who wrote "Malignant Sadness"), wrote a beautiful little book as a primer for teaching scientific understanding, entitled "The Un-natural Nature of Science". That precisely is the point. Science is all about falsifying your theories, it is counter-intuitive and a completely un-natural way of viewing the world.

So what can be the evolutionary advantage for a belief in the supernatural?

I had been puzzling over this for sometime when a close friend of mine Dr. Howard Hershon, a distinguished psychiatrist, provided the answer over a game of bridge. He argues this way: The bigger the tribe the more successful. With greater muscle the tribe can conquer neighbours, take more wives and cultivate more land. However this depends on having powerful leadership. A chieftain emerges who might be very clever or very strong in armed combat. He will reign supreme until he weakens or other alpha males start competing. This system then has inbuilt instability that might be described with mathematical chaos theory. Sooner or later the tribe will fragment into warring factions and be at risk of conquest by the neighbours. On the other hand if their leader is a supernatural, omniscient and omnipotent being, then the tribe can only grow because no one can defeat their king.

In evolutionary terms one might expect homo-scientificus, who emerged at the Age of Enlightenment, to outpace and dominate homo-sapiens; after all, look at the fruits of scientific discovery; longer healthier lives, faster transport and instant world wide communication. Yet the scientific gene has built in the seeds of its own destruction.

The fruits of science are available to all; the technological offspring of scientific discovery are available to all, which means the weapons of mass destruction (WMD) are available to all! If WMD get into the hands of un-evolved homo-sapiens and they wish to take over the world, in the name of their great and invisible chieftain, then G*D save us all!

Chapter 18

The Limits of Science;
Arts and Humanities

Two years ahead of my 65th birthday I took early retirement from the NHS in order to save my sanity before the Alice in Wonderland world of "joined up management" drove me into another acute depressive illness. Without dwelling too much on these unfortunate times one simple vignette will suffice to explain what we, the consultant staff, had to put up with. Within the same month I received two directives. Firstly I was advised that no patient diagnosed or suspected of breast cancer should have to wait more than two weeks for surgery; perfectly fine by me. Next I learnt that one of my operating lists was to be withdrawn as I was "over performing"! That is management jargon for carrying out more life saving operations than had been purchased in advance by our local primary health care trust. Furthermore I still had to cancel booked admissions at the last minute because there were no beds available even to allow me to occupy one operating list. When the deputy complaints manager asked me to account for myself and explain why I wasn't fulfilling my contract I took it as nature's way of telling me to get out alive. It's worth mentioning in passing that after more than 40 years loyal service to the NHS my departure went unmarked without even a tea party or a long service watch and chain. I therefore decided to limit myself to a modest private practice in the West End, but continued to teach. As I no longer had access to patients in the NHS wards of the Middlesex and University College Hospitals I gave up teaching surgery and diverted my energies to teaching the emerging new discipline of "Medical Humanities".

Having stressed the importance of science in medicine in this book

208

so far this chapter serves to emphasize my views of the role of the humanities as a balance. It also will serve to illustrate the futility of trying to separate the "two cultures" in the practice of clinical medicine where one should buttress the other like the two columns of an arch with the patient as the keystone.

Amongst the many German doctors indicted at Nuremberg for crimes against humanity in 1946 were tenured professors, clinical directors, personal physicians, the head of the German Red Cross and bio-medical researchers employed by the pharmaceutical industry. Some of the leading physicians amongst Germany's medical establishment even committed suicide before their interrogation or indictment. Many of these were considered men of refined culture and the music of Wagner and Beethoven was often broadcast over the loudspeakers in the concentration camps. It can thus be seen that culture alone does not make for a humane physician and the function of the arts and humanities in the training of doctors is not to enjoy a night at the opera when they qualify, but to ensure that they make better and more humane physicians who are instinctively appalled by human suffering and do everything within their power, even to the point of significant self-sacrifice to save a life or to succour someone in mortal pain.

During my time as a medical educator I've witnessed the ever-expanding knowledge base that we try to impose on our students with an ever-worsening ratio of staff-to-student numbers. The developments of cell and molecular biology which impact on all human disease processes is taking an increasing share of our curriculum time with the ever-present danger that molecular reductionism may somehow leave the whole patient behind. Yet as a clinician and a scientist I want to resist falling into the popular trap of post-modern relativism in rejecting the scientific method in favour of some vague metaphysical notion of "holistic" medicine.

At the same time I share a view with many of my senior academic colleagues that there is a real danger of losing the humanity in the practice of medicine by ignoring many of the subjects that are conventionally taught within the Faculty of Humanities. I believe with great fervour that the teaching of arts and humanities, in addition to ensuring that our young doctors practice in an ethical and humane way, will paradoxically enhance their understanding of science and improve their communication skills; thus transforming them into better diagnosticians, whilst improving the satisfaction of their patient clients.

Science and the Arts are the twin pillars upon which our Western cultural heritage are supported, yet little progress has been made since CP Snow's seminal essays of the 1960s demonstrated the separation of these two cultures. The polarization of these two bodies of knowledge is perpetuated by our education system to the impoverishment of all. Even the best educated amongst our political and academic leaders have lost close on 50% of their cultural inheritance and the Renaissance man has all but disappeared from modern society.

Yet before we get carried away in our derogation of the scientist let us remember that the members of the arts faculties are equally illiterate in the understanding of science. It is therefore fair to quote the following passage from an essay by Melvyn Bragg, "it is impossible to be educated today in an advanced society and confess to a lack of knowledge or interest in science; It is obvious to me that scientists know far more about the arts than arts people know about the sciences"

The spectacular advances over the last two decades in the development of recombinant technology, the decoding of the human genome, and the technology of molecular research, has contributed to the advancement of science, yet has deconstructed the human subject to a molecular level. Inevitably better understanding of human disease and better treatments will emerge from this process and in itself I have no argument against this degree of reductionism. Unfortunately, we have so far been unable to reconstitute the complex organism of the human being up through the various hierarchical levels to that of a successful and healthy personality existing comfortably within his own society. I think it is an exaggeration to argue that this reductionism resulting from molecular biology has led to the brutalisation of medicine, but certainly it has done nothing to contribute to the humanisation of our subject.

Paradoxically when treatments were least effective the humanitarian instinct of the doctor was virtually all that was on offer. You have only got to read the romance of "Dr Finlay's Case Book" to appreciate what was no doubt an approximation to this truth. Yet as treatments become more effective and the pace of change is likely to increase within the next millennium, doctors are in danger of losing their humanitarian instincts to become mere technocrats, often expressing a conceit in their wish to medicalize aspects of human behaviour which are strictly none of the doctors' business.

I believe that the Arts-Science dichotomy in the practice of Medicine is entirely fallacious as both are integral to the skilled practice of modern medicine. I say this not out of political correctness (I am most certainly not "touchy-feely") but out of a hard-nosed pragmatic view based on over 30 years experience as a clinical scientist.

I would briefly like to discuss the practical applications of philosophy, theology, literature/theatre, fine art and music for the enhancement of medical education.

Philosophy and Theology in Relation to the Understanding and Teaching of Medical Ethics

Medical ethics are not absolute codes of conduct that leapt fully formed and immutable from the heads of ancient sages in distant times. Medical ethics in fact demonstrate an uncomfortable plasticity with subtle variations emerging between different ages in history and between different ethnic and cultural groups. Medical ethics may be driven by the law of the land or by medical technology, but more often than not medical technology runs in advance of our capacity for ethical control and the law is a blunt instrument that may belatedly react to some of the worst medical abuses or as a late reaction to public outcry. All ethical codes of conduct for the practice of medicine have their bedrock in philosophy and theology. For example, the Hippocratic oath, which is seldom recited today, probably emerged as a result of the teachings of respect for human rights and dignity at the time of democracy in Athens 400 BCE. Much of the teaching of Plato and Socrates can be seen reflected in the teachings of Hippocrates. In contrast, contemporary medical ethics are heavily dependent on the teachings of Immanuel Kant of the 19th Century AD and his four "categorical imperatives" – autonomy, beneficence, non-maleficence and justice. If only it was that easy! Contemporary medical problems illustrate the tensions that arise when there is often a clash of these categorical imperatives, particularly between distributive justice on one hand and the right to autonomy or self-determination on the other. Furthermore, some of these "categorical imperatives" clash with ethnic or religious minorities. For example, an absolute belief in the right to self-determination would encourage suicide and assisted euthanasia, which would be an anathema to orthodox Jewish teaching. The Jewish faith believes that life is of infinite value and you cannot split infinity. Therefore every moment of life is of infinite value, and therefore the individual or the doctor working on the individual's instruction must not do anything to shorten life. In a similar way, witness the furore regarding the debate between the anti-abortionist (who describe themselves as pro-lifers) and those demanding the freedom of the individual to control their families by the use of abortion where necessary (pro-choice). According to Roman Catholic doctrine, life begins at conception and the individual does not have sufficient autonomy to end the life of the unborn child. Thus, even within our narrow Western world of Judeo-Christian belief system, there are many tensions. Yet when we recognise that our society exhibits an enormous range of cultural and religious diversity, the problems are magnified. For example, how do we accommodate the shariah law of Islam and the Hindu systems of caste and belief in reincarnation? Once again we are in danger of losing respect for minorities within our pluralistic society, whilst on the other hand drifting guiltily into the relativistic political aspiration of multiculturism that implies "anything goes". Our young doctors must learn to respect and celebrate the ethnic and cultural diversity of the society in which they work, and therefore need to study the fundamentals of theological belief shared by large numbers of their prospective patients.

Of course, theology plays a much more important role in society than merely underpinning our code of medical ethics. Theology is the basis of faith and faith provides spiritual solace for our patients at the time of suffering and when confronting the inevitability of death. The practice of religion can contribute to the healing of the spirit, but a clear demarcation has to be made from spiritual healing and healing of the body, although we must leave room to speculate on the links that might exist between a spirit at peace with itself and a body best equipped to heal itself. Nevertheless, from my own experience in oncology, I must warn my students of the quackery which finds fertile soil in filling the gaps vacated by faith in an essentially secular society. The "new age" belief systems have led to a return to animism, idolatry, witchcraft, astrology and the magic bough. It is no exaggeration that the magic bough (mistletoe) is demonstrating a remarkable reincarnation as Iscador, one of the most popular "unproven" remedies for the treatment of advanced cancer.

Literature and Theatre

The study of literature and theatre might have three important roles in the education of doctors; rebuilding medical idealism, deflating medical pomposity and providing us with a window into personal suffering.

It distressed me recently to learn that none of my students at University College London had read Axel Munthe's "The Story of San Michele" or A.J. Cronin's "The Citadel". For my generation of medical students these wonderful stories fuelled our idealism, and there was no sense of shame in admitting at the interview for medical school entrance that you wished to become a doctor out of idealism and a wish to serve humanity.

In contrast, the inhumane pompous and arrogant doctor who inevitably gets his comeuppance has been beautifully satirized in the works of Voltaire or George Bernard Shaw. I would like to recommend that all medical students read the preface to "The Doctor's Dilemma" as well as the play itself. The Sir Ralph Bloomfield Bonnington character, satirized by Shaw, still exists amongst the higher echelons of the medical establishment, but sadly we also see these attitudes amongst young doctors who know all about molecular biology on the one hand and the commissioning of services on the other, but little about the feelings of the patient in the middle! Perhaps one of the best lessons in medical humility is to study the history of our subject and recognize that most of our added years and reduction in infant mortality has nothing to do with medicine but all to do with improvements in public health and the relief of poverty. It was as much a result of the righteous indignation of idealistic politicians after reading the 19th C novels of Charles Dickens, as anything achieved by doctors in that time, that contributed to improvements in the welfare of infants and young children. This same sense of righteous indignation should be experienced by medical students reading some of the wonderful contemporary novels emerging from the Indian sub-continent or by first-hand experience doing electives in the developing world, getting out into the slums instead of spending time on Pattaya beach. This recognition of the impact of social injustice on health will then educate the young doctor in the true meaning of the ethics of distributive justice, health economics and the inevitability of rationing. It is the politician's right and responsibility to decide on what proportion of the Gross National Product should be allocated to welfare, housing or medicine. It is then left to the medical establishment to apportion their share of the cake to public health measures, primary health care or high technology medicine in the acute sector. The allocation of scarce resources within a just and humane society demands the recognition that our most precious resource is skilled manpower, who then have to make decisions such as the allocation of funding. If more is to be spent on organ transplantations, for example, then less will be available for the not so glamorous pursuits such as the care of the elderly, the chronically infirm or the mentally ill.

Literature and the theatre also provide us with a window on personal suffering. We often talk about empathizing with our patients, but this is a meaningless cliché without a genuine understanding of the fears and suffering of our patients. A pre-requisite for sensitive doctoring demands good communication skills that are dependent on genuine empathy, and the gift of listening. We should also exploit our patient's natural gift for story telling. We should teach our students patience in listening to the anecdotes of old soldiers and old sailors who were provided with free tobacco during the Second World War and then subsequently admitted with gangrene of their lower limbs to our modern high-tech hospitals. Students should respect the gift of story-telling and not be confined to the straitjacket of the conventional history taking. Taken to extreme, an individuals' experience of disease and suffering linked with a lyrical gift of poetry, literature and the transcendental can produce the most beautiful and moving prose. For example Julia Rose, one of the most promising philosophers of our age, had her life cut short by cancer and published a book shortly before her diagnosis entitled "Love's Work". It is extremely moving to read this passage with the knowledge of what was awaiting her. "*I would like to pass unnoticed which is why I hope that I am not deprived of old age, I aspire to a Miss Marple persona, to be exactly as I am, decrepit nature, yet supernature in one, equally alert on the damp ground and in the turbulent air. Perhaps I don't have to wait for old age for that invisible trespass and pedestrian tread. Insensible of mortality and desperately mortal*".

The History and Execution of Fine Art

Doctors, in addition to being interested in the history of art, are often gifted amateur artists, and this trait is seen commonly amongst surgeons of the highest rank. For them art can be a therapy releasing them from the frustrations, tensions and anxieties of their day to day work by exercising the other half of the brain.

But it is at this point that we stray into the territory of art as therapy, which is not strictly our remit. Yet my experience in being an advocate for art therapy in my years at the Royal Marsden Hospital exposed me to the intense imagery provided by even the least gifted patient, providing them with a catharsis and us with an insight or a window into their suffering and fear. In many ways this is analogous to the role of literature, but in the case of art, all patients are able to express themselves even with the most naïve of images, whereas few are sufficiently gifted to express themselves in writing.

Some time in 1990, shortly after I was appointed Professor of Surgery at the RMH, I was making a solitary ward round, checking on the welfare of my breast cancer patients, when I came upon an unfamiliar woman handing out pots of paint to a patient recovering from my surgical assault. Assuming she was an occupational therapist and wanting to make my presence felt, I engaged her in conversation. Within five minutes of talking to Camilla Connell, I was totally won over to the concept of art therapy for patients with cancer. Since that day, a warm relationship has developed between us, based on mutual respect and understanding for the contributions we can each make to patients recovering from cancer surgery, or for that matter, any other life-threatening disorder.

My interest and enthusiasm can be described at two levels. First, there is an uncanny thematic similarity running through the works of many of these patients who face serious disease. It is as if the experience of cancer stimulates some deeply hidden communal memory to evoke the symbolism of life and death, fear and hope. The tree, for example, is a recurring theme in these works of art, one that can be traced back through many cultures to the original *etz chaim* (tree of life) of the Old Testament. (Figures 55, 56, 57)

At an individual level, what I have found so moving is the obvious cathartic value of using art to express hidden fears, the progression of the imagery from fear to hope as a sign of recovery and sadly, in the reverse direction, as a sign of deterioration. There is no doubt that art is a powerful medium for self-expression for frightened patients who do not have the words or the will to express themselves verbally.

Many patients have hidden talents, yet even in the absence of conventional artistic skill some of their almost childlike and naïve pictures are enormously expressive and deeply moving to the observer. I believe that art therapy is a unique vehicle for allowing patients with cancer to express hidden emotions and thus, to some extent, provide their own psychotherapy.

As a practical expression of my enthusiasm and support I helped Camilla organize an exhibition of the patients' art that was shown first at the Royal Marsden Hospital and then continued as a peripatetic exhibition around medical centres in the UK. I also used my authority to help raise funding for a second part-time art therapist to work at the Sutton branch of our institution.

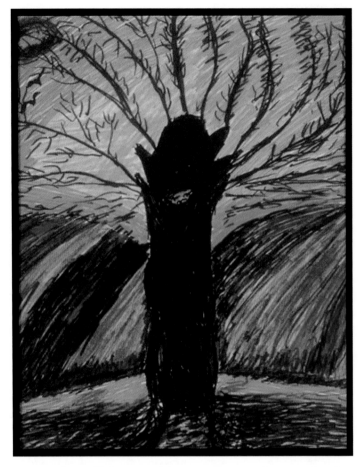

Fig. 55 Tree of life painted by a woman just diagnosed with breast cancer

Whilst this was going on, the Marsden, like other cancer centres in London, was facing closure as a result of the Tomlinson Report on the future of London hospital services. As Professor of Surgery and Director of Clinical Research, I was placed in the front line of the battle to save the hospital. This was also at a time when planning blight led to the early retirement of one of my consultant colleagues and departure of another for a different teaching hospital. I was left to run the department virtually single-handed.

The stress of this workload and our uncertain future were almost too much to bear. I placed myself at Camilla's mercy to provide art therapy for my own struggle. I elected to undertake private tuition in

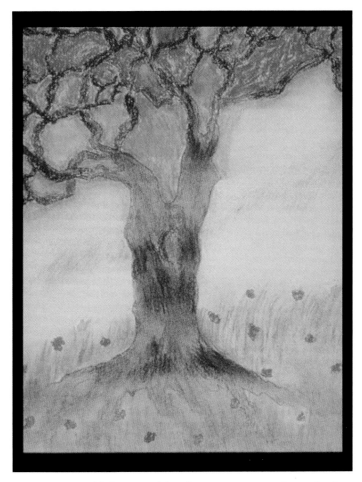

Fig. 56 Tree of life painted by the same woman 6 months later

portrait sculpture (which is her particular expertise). I learnt at first hand the benefits of self-expression through the medium of clay. The journey through a lifeless lump of material to a recognizable portrait of my daughter was sufficiently cathartic to help me cope with my struggles (I suspect that some of my fiercest attacks on the clay were surrogates for physical abuse of the bureaucrats who were trying to destroy the wonderful institution of the Royal Marsden Hospital).

I therefore have both first and second hand experience of the power of art therapy. I acknowledge that this is anecdotal evidence, and as a clinical scientist I would not accept art therapy on these merits alone – but I truly believe that it has a part to play in the management of

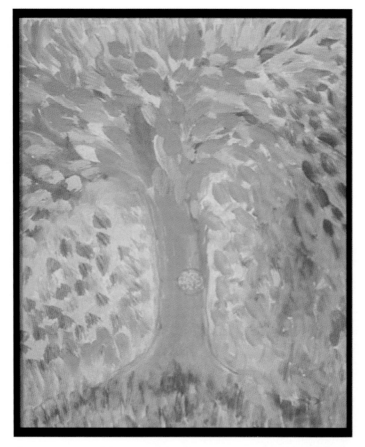

Fig. 57 Tree of life painted by the same woman a year after diagnosis

the sick and the frightened, and that it is also a topic suitable for scientific evaluation using established instruments for the monitoring of a patient's quality of life.

Good medicine is not only the practice of the science of the subject, but also the practice of the humanities of the subject. Central to the humanitarian practice of medicine is the development of good communication skills. Central to the development of good communication skills is the development of empathy. Strictly, empathy means trying to get inside the patient's head, to feel his or her fears and pain, a task that even the most empathetic of doctors can find extremely difficult. As far as I am concerned, art therapy is the most direct line into the patient's experience of illness, and I feel almost ashamed that I do not make use of it in the day to day practice of my own clinic. Perhaps there simply are not enough Camilla Connells to go round. If there were, I have little doubt that the drugs budget for the NHS would fall, as prescriptions for anxyolitics and anti-depressants would be replaced by the prescription of art therapy.

The traditional link between art and medicine has been in the illustration of anatomy texts, and more recently the illustrations in textbooks, in particular for the techniques of complex surgical procedures. Perhaps the most famous textbook of anatomy of all time was published by Vesalius in the 16th century and illustrated by Stephan van Calcar, one of Titian's ablest pupils. (Figure 58)

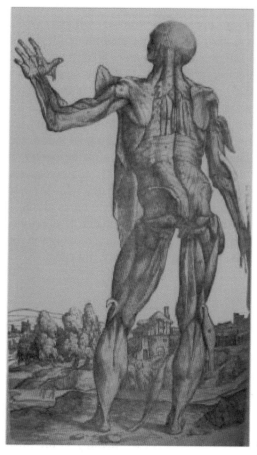

Fig. 58 Anatomical drawing from Vesalius' textbook

219

Art is also a very powerful teaching medium. Wittingly, or unwittingly, great artists of the past have been skilled at illustrating the ravages of disease and deformity, and this has been a subject of fascination for artists and doctors alike in the last few decades. For example, Masaccio's cripple illustrated in one of his frescoes of the Brancacci chapel in Florence or the goiter of Dante Gabriel Rossetti's favourite model. My personal favourite is the inadvertent illustration of breast cancer in Rembrandt's moving painting of Bathsheba at her toilet in the Louvre Museum as I described in the earlier chapter on the natural history of breast cancer.

Another direction that could be pursued is the way physical handicap might impact on artists and their creativity. A recent illustration concerned Monet's cataracts as described in The Lancet of December 1996. One could argue whether the cataracts contributed to his creativity as suggested by the author of the piece, or in my opinion that the maturation of any artist with or without visual impairment can improve on creativity. The same enigma applies to El Greco's paintings with their astigmatic appearance. Historians of art, who argue that the visual defect contributed to El Greco's perception, have obviously overlooked the logical solecism of this interpretation. Renoir's rheumatoid arthritis meant that he had to paint with his brushes strapped to his wrist, and yet this if anything enhanced the quality of his work, and Aubrey Beardsley's fevered imagination was fuelled by his tuberculosis. There are many parallels to the poetry of John Keats who also died at a tragically young age from tuberculosis. It is also worth reading biographies of Aubrey Beardsley who frittered away the last couple of years of his life chasing miracle cures amongst the watering holes of Europe. In fact the whole subject of creativity and disease has been covered in a beautiful short monograph by Professor Philip Sandbolm of Gothenburg University, Sweden.

Musical Performance and Appreciation

Exactly as with painting, music can be therapy for the doctor as well as the patient, either in its performance or in its appreciation. Many physicians are amateur musicians and no doubt enjoy a release from the tensions of being a doctor when performing. And to discuss music as therapy is once again outside my remit.

There is a fascinating linkage between the appreciation of music and of speech, and yet there are paradoxical relationships between aphasia and amusia. Oliver Sacks, a physician with the gift of an accomplished writer, describes many such examples from his experience, and in particular in his delightful book of short anecdotes "The Man Who Mistook His Wife For A Hat". There are patients with severe mental or neurological disabilities who are capable of appreciating or performing music at the highest levels. As with art, the great composers have suffered disease that has affected their physical and mental well-being, which inevitably has had an influence on their creativity. Once again this subject is covered in Philip Sandblom's monograph or more recently in Anton Neumayr's book, "Music and Medicine". In parallel with my discussion about artists and their perception, one could discuss the impact of Beethoven's deafness and the creativity of his latter years alongside Monet's cataracts and his perception of the House of Commons at twilight.

At this point I would like to briefly mention opera. The opera is a remarkable amalgam of theatre, design, spectacle and music, but inevitably one has to ask the awkward question "do the death scenes of Mimi and Violetta in La Boheme and La Traviata add pathos or bathos to terminal tuberculosis?" This delicate balance depends heavily on the sensitivity of the director, which is another aspect of the performing arts. The Doctor as Director has a fine tradition and of course the leading contemporary exponent is Dr Jonathan Miller.

It is hoped that the student of tomorrow may be drawn towards some of these other disciplines and that opportunities to study for example a language or to undertake a project related to literature or the history of medicine, may be offered. In the meantime each individual clinical teacher can make a start by introducing these subjects into the day-to-day teaching on his under-graduate firm. I will illustrate how this can be achieved without any additional cost, without making any additional demands on the curriculum, but making extra demands of our medical students who will see this as a labour of love, rather than an additional chore.

****

I teach surgery. I have always taught surgery. I have a specialist interest in cancer so much of my teaching involves oncology. Much of the time that my medical students spend on "the Firm" is involved in witnessing and learning simple practical tasks. My students lose much sleep, taking it in turns to be on call with the junior medical staff dealing with surgical emergencies. My students have an in-course assessment and have to pass a final exam in surgery in order to qualify. You might therefore think that this is the most unpromising environment for the introduction in even a limited way of the teaching of medical humanities. This is simply not the case and I wish to illustrate this in two ways; firstly by describing my introductory seminar to each new group of students on the Firm and secondly by the teaching of narrative as an integral component of the conventional teaching of history taking and communication skills which apply equally well to surgical patients as to any other discipline.

At the start of each Firm I select a patient currently under my care and illustrate by example how to prepare and present a case history. I then go on to dissect the individual case to ask the question, "how can the study of arts and humanities help this patient and his or her family?" Let me provide you with an example.

****

Mrs Sarah G – 29 years old

- *This young woman is asymptomatic but presented to my clinic following the detection of a suspicious abnormality on mammographic screening. Fine needle aspiration cytology was suspicious of breast cancer.*

- *There is no relevant past medical history and she is gravid 1 para 1*

- *There is a significant family medical history. She is of Ashkenasi Jewish origin. Her mother died of breast cancer at the age of 36 and her sister was recently diagnosed with bilateral breast cancer at the age of 21. A paternal aunt had breast cancer at the age of 37.*

- *On clinical examination she was a fit young woman and the only abnormality of note was an area of ill-defined nodularity in the upper outer quadrant of her right breast.*

- *Special investigations were reviewed. The mammograms which she had for screening because of her family history showed an area of microcalcifications in the upper outer quadrant of the right breast. Fine needle aspiration cytology showed atypical cells but a core cut biopsy showed duct carcinoma in situ and also areas of invasive duct cancer of intermediate grade.*

- *In the interval between diagnosis and the planning of surgery, the patient mentioned that she had missed a period and pregnancy testing was positive.*

- *How should this patient be treated and what should we do about her pregnancy?*

****

How can the study of arts and humanities help Sarah and her family? The simple stereotype way by which I present the case history was intentional. Nothing but the patient's true narrative of her own life experience and fears can do justice to this story. We must recognize that her mother died young and as a result she was brought up by an aunt. We must recognize what it must feel like to be forced to come to terms with one's mortality at such an early age and the clinical history alone cannot do justice to the strength of feeling of Sarah and her husband about producing a sibling for their little daughter, in other words the pregnancy is very precious.

By allowing the patient to provide her own narrative, this indirectly enhances the communication skills of the student and helps them develop empathy and rapport. Much of good communication skills depends on the doctor being a good listener and patient satisfaction can often be enhanced when they recognize that the doctor is listening and by listening paying respect.

Next we come to the major ethical issues that are raised by this case. From her family tree and Ashkenasi origins it is highly likely that there is a germ line mutation in the BRCA1 or BRCA2 gene. Sarah had already been counselled on this matter, hence her exposure to mammographic screening, yet she had opted not to go forward for the genetic test because at the time there was no proven intervention, if she would have tested positive. Now her own cancer has made it even more likely that this extended family has a germ line mutation, putting increasing pressure on other female relatives for genetic testing. This leads on to a further consideration of the genotype of the foetus. Would she want to know if it was male or female and abort the female, might it be possible to test for the gene on a cell of the developing foetus if a female and abort the female foetus if the test is positive? Unfortunately our ethical guidelines on these difficult issues are falling far behind the rapid pace of progress at the molecular level.

Next the issue of abortion itself: Is this ethical or unethical? Well this of course depends very much on the cultural and religious background of her family. In a largely secular society most patients would consider themselves rational humanists and therefore feel that they should be fully autonomous in this decision. Yet as already described if the patient was Catholic then abortion would be considered a sin whereas, according to the Jewish faith if the abortion would prolong her life, by even a day, then it might be considered an ethical imperative to proceed with the abortion. This immediately brings us back to the issue of epistemology. Although in theory it is plausible that the continuation of the pregnancy may increase the rate of progression of her breast cancer, are there empirical data that support or refute that opinion? In fact the weight of evidence would suggest that if anything women with breast cancer who become pregnant have a better outcome than expected, once again illustrating the beauty of the deductive logic whereby a plausible hypothesis is overturned by the accumulation of empirical data. Whilst on the subject of epistemology we then have to consider the evidence for and against different treatment modalities in this case and also be in a position to weigh up the balance between quality of life and length of life, as a result of these different treatments. It so happens we have an enormous weight of evidence that will help Sarah with her decision-making process about treatment. We know with confidence that conservative surgery supplemented by radiotherapy will provide the same chance of cure as more radical surgery. We now know that adjuvant systemic chemotherapy in young women with breast cancer significantly prolongs life but what about the effect of chemotherapy on the foetus? Again it is plausible that chemotherapy may have such an adverse effect on the unborn child that in order to provide the patient with the best chance of survival the foetus should be aborted, yet empirical data suggest that once organogenesis is complete, the unborn child is remarkably robust and can in fact tolerate chemotherapy. I have often cared for patients, throughout their pregnancy, whilst treating their breast cancer, ably supported by a team of clinical oncologists, medical oncologists and gynaecologists. So if the continuation of her pregnancy is not likely to interfere with treatment and thus impair her length of life and if the foetus is tolerant of the treatment, then the only matter left to consider for this precious pregnancy is the possibility of Sarah dying young, leaving a second orphaned child to be brought up by Sarah's husband.

This to me was the most difficult component of managing this case and it comes back to the ethical problems of truth telling. However painful it was for me as a personal physician, I felt that it was my responsibility to inform Sarah and her husband that breast cancer at the age of 29 has a very poor prognosis and whilst supporting their wish to continue with the pregnancy they needed to be aware of the dreadful possibility that the baby would be left without a mother; but then as Sarah reminded me she also grew up without a mother and her life to date has been fulfilled, whilst her husband's response demonstrated a nobility of spirit. He was prepared to shoulder the burden with the compensation that there would always be two sets of eyes to remind him of his beautiful wife. You can easily imagine how that interview ended up with tears all round and even this rough\ tough bloodthirsty surgeon had to cover his face with a handkerchief whilst simulating a bout of sneezing.

Finally facing an uncertain future coming to terms with her own mortality Sarah needed spiritual and psychological support which was certainly beyond my own competence or even that of my nurse counsellor. In addition to her extended family and her Jewish faith we were able to call upon the agency of Chai-Lifeline, a volunteer organization set up specifically to work alongside doctors in this difficult and sensitive area.

Whatever the sub-specialty any under-graduate teaching Firm is the ideal setting for the teaching of narrative, and through narrative enhance the communication skills of the students, their capacity to listen and their capacity to empathize. However I take the subject one step forward by actively encouraging my students to collect the patient's narrative and write them up as a piece of literature, encouraging them to draw on all their skills and enthusiasms that antedated their entry into medical school and which like any other talent atrophies with disuse. To further help and encourage them in this endeavour I insist that they read literature outside their medical textbooks and promise them that this then becomes the labour of love. Faith McLellan and Ann Hudson-Jones, both from the Institute of Medical Humanities at the University of Texas, Galveston, have written much on the importance of the study of literature by medical students and Ann Hudson-Jones has described an evolving canon of literature that will enhance the students' understanding of the experience of ill health.

****

One Sunday evening in December a few years back my wife and I went to the Barbican to listen to Verdi's Requiem. The interior architecture and the gold ochre of the paneling produced an immediate sense of peace and tranquility. The music and poetry of the piece eloquently describe the fear of death, the terror of the Day of Judgment, yet the optimism and faith in a rebirth of the spirit. For example, the verses 2–5 of the sequence with the extraordinary trumpeting from the brass section that makes the hair on the back of your scalp stand on end, says it all "*quantus tremor est futures…. How great a terror there will be when the Judge shall come, he who shall examine all things strictly – the trumpet spreading its wondrous sound to the tombs of the whole world, will bring everyone before the throne. Death and nature shall be dumbfounded when creation rises again to answer its Judge*". Finally in the last section, Agnus Dei the words of solace, and the change from the minor to the major key, allow you to leave the auditorium with your despair replaced by euphoria and optimism. The experience might be even more sublime if you also happen to be of the Christian faith, they seem to have better tunes than my lot!

Either way, Verdi has enriched the life of many, including myself, and I would like to think my patients find me a more amiable and tolerant doctor on a Monday morning than I would otherwise be without his help.

Chapter 19

Does Breast Cancer Exist in a State of Chaos? Towards a new Paradigm of the Disease

Valentine " *We're better at predicting events at the edge of the galaxy or inside the nucleus of the atom than whether it will rain on auntie's garden party three Sunday's from now.... We can't even predict the next drip from a dripping tap when it gets irregular. Each drip sets up conditions for the next, the smallest variation blows predictions apart, and the weather is unpredictable the same way, will always be unpredictable ... It's the best possible time to be alive, when almost everything you thought you knew is wrong."*

Tom Stoppard, Arcadia Act 1 scene 4.

Just over 10 years ago I went with my wife and a couple of friends to see the first production of Tom Stoppard's new play, Arcadia, at the National Theatre. Towards the end of the first act the character Valentine Coverly, a Cambridge mathematician, came up with the words quoted above. He was trying to explain his excitement about the new mathematics of chaos theory to his fiancée Hannah Jarvis. When I listened to his speech I experienced a "eureka" moment that

I tried to share with my company without much success. I had been mulling over certain discrepancies in Fisher's model of breast cancer that had guided my research up until that point. If the facts don't fit the model then the model is wrong, not the other way round. Furthermore as Thomas Huxley, Darwin's great friend, once said; "The great tragedy of science – the slaying of a beautiful hypothesis by an ugly fact." For a more up to date take on this I would refer readers to "The Black Swan; the Impact of the Highly Improbable" by Nassim Nicholas Taleb. The "black swan" according to Taleb is; "...an *outlier*, as it lies outside the realm of regular expectations.... it carries an extreme impact and in spite of its outlier status, human nature makes us concoct explanations for its occurrence *after* the fact, making it explainable and predictable". However hard I try I simply can't make the natural history of breast cancer predictable because, like Valentine's weather systems, the behaviour of breast cancer is for the most part unpredictable. If that is the case then we are using the wrong mathematical equations, the disease doesn't follow linear systems but non-linear or chaos mathematics. Professor Sir Robert May, one of this country's greatest mathematical thinkers, put it this way in the programme notes for the 2009 production of Arcadia at the Duke of York's Theatre; "Now we realise that extraordinary complex behaviour can be generated by the simplest rules. It seems likely to me that much complexity and apparent irregularity seen in nature, from the development of individual creatures to the structure of eco-systems, derives from simple – but chaotic – rules." After that eureka moment I contacted Robert May who was at the time President of the Royal Society. He put me in touch with an ex PhD student of his, Mark Chaplain of the University of Dundee, and together with him and a few like minded chums, we eventually published a paper in the European Journal of Cancer in 2004 entitled, "Does breast cancer exist in a state of chaos?" The mathematical equation that we came up with produced a three dimensional image of a growth on the computer screen which perfectly mimicked the real thing. (http://www.maths.dundee.ac.uk/~chaplain/tumour_fig4.gif)

I now wish to describe some of the logical inconsistencies, the black swans, which provoked this attack of insanity.

If we believe that once a primary tumour gains access to the vasculature it starts seeding metastases (secondary tumours) in a linear or exponential manner, it should be expected that because a larger tumour has been in the body for a longer time, and therefore has had access to the vasculature for longer than smaller tumours, a much higher percentage of patients with larger tumours should present with metastases. This is true to some extent with regard to lymphatic metastases, i.e. there is a correlation of the number of involved lymph nodes with the size of the primary tumour. However, this relationship is far from linear. Thus there are small or even occult tumours that have several involved lymph nodes involved, while many large tumours are found not to have metastasized to the axilla. This discrepancy becomes even more apparent when we consider *distant* metastases. It would be expected that the proportion of patients presenting with distant metastases would be higher for those with larger tumours as opposed to those with smaller tumours. Nevertheless, in real life a patient presenting with a primary tumour along with distant metastases is uncommon, however large the tumour. In fact, the percentages of patients that present with symptomatic metastases is 0%, 3% and 7% in stages I, II and III of the primary tumour, respectively. However, when you look at the incidence of metastases in these same groups 18 months after their primary diagnosis and *surgery*, there is a clear correlation of primary tumour size with the proportion of patients experiencing distant relapse. (About 5% for stage I and 25% for stage III)

How can this be explained without challenging the linear model of breast cancer spread? One explanation would be that although the number of metastases that are seeded by the primary tumour would be linearly related to the tumour size and biological aggressiveness, the clinical appearance of metastases is triggered or accelerated only after the primary tumour has been disturbed or removed. This conclusion may logically derive from a consideration of the pessimistic experiences of ancient surgeons I described in chapter 4. It also is the result of very modern day science using computer simulations to analyze an unexpected bimodal hazard rate of relapse for patients treated only with surgical excision of primary breast tumours. Hazards are calculated by dividing the number of events in a particular time frame by the number of patients at risk of having those events at the start of the period. This is an important way of looking at data because it emphasizes when adverse events occur rather than just the cumulative result. Since no one lives forever, including breast cancer patients, **when** the increased risk for recurrence and death occur is more important than the cumulative risk. (Figure 59)

I have to conclude that the majority of metastases at the time of diagnosis are dormant rather than actively growing. What is the nature of this dormancy? Within the dormant metastasis there is balance

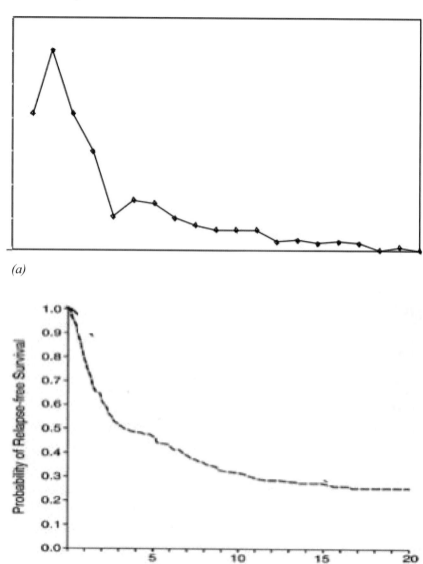

(a)

(b)

Fig. 59 *Hazard rate and actuarial plot of the same data set. a) Shows when the adverse events are likely to occur and b) shows the cumulative effect*

between cell growth and cell death. This is partly determined by factors that inhibit blood vessel development (angiogenesis) without which a clump of cancer cells can't grow more than 10^{8-9} (i.e. the size of a pin head) and other factors that stimulate angiogenesis. To maintain a dormant state, inhibiting factors locally dominate. If stimulating factors are increased or inhibiting factors are reduced the dormant condition can no longer be maintained. In other words this dormancy isn't like sleep, it is a system in a state of dynamic equilibrium.

It is well documented in animal models that removal of the primary tumour will reduce the inhibition of angiogenesis and it is known that after surgery a sharp spike in angiogenesis stimulators and growth factors occurs to aid in wound healing. Thus it is not surprising that tumour angiogenesis and proliferation result after surgery to remove the primary cancer. Thus a likely trigger for 'kick-starting' the growth of dormant metastases could be the act of surgery itself.

After surgery for breast cancer the first peak in the incidence of secondary disease occurs at two to three years, the same time, whether the tumour was at stage I or stage III. It is only the amplitude of the peak that changes with stage, the later the stage the higher is the peak, but the timing of the signal remains the same.

These phenomena suggest a nonlinear dynamic model for breast cancer, which, like a chaotic system, is exquisitely sensitive to events around the time of diagnosis. It suggests that surgery could be responsible for accelerating the clinical appearance of metastatic disease.

Clearly a new model for breast cancer is needed that takes into account the fine dynamic balance between the tumour and the host, including various biological signalling factors which influence cell proliferation, cell death and angiogenesis. At this point I joined forces with three other experts who shared my views, Romano Demicheli from the Department of Medical Oncology, Istituto Nazionale dei Tumori, Milan, Mike Retsky from the Department of Vascular Biology, Children's Hospital and Harvard Medical School, Boston, and William Hrushesky from The University of South Carolina, Columbia, USA.

Taking all this into account we went on to develop a new model to explain the natural history of the disease which, in addition to explaining the success of the Fisherian model of "biological predeterminism", also explained the clinical observations from antiquity that fail to fit neatly into the contemporary early detection paradigm. (see chapter 17)

The conclusion that more surgery is better is similar to the conclusion that earlier detection/earlier therapy is better. This linear thinking has however not served us well. The reaction of Halsted's disciples was simply to assume that surgery had to encompass a greater field. The reaction of the mammographic screening community has been identical, calling for earlier and more frequent examinations. Neither radical surgery nor earlier screening-induced surgery are, however, free of harm. This linear thinking has done more harm than good. This is because the host-cancer-surgery interaction is not linear.

First of all cancer should be seen as a process, not a morphological entity. Individual cancers, while likely to originate from single cells, are constantly adapting to the local environment. There is no single substance or metabolic defect that is unique to cancer. The cancer cell is largely normal, both genetically and functionally. The malignant properties are the result of a small number of genetic and/or environmental changes that have a profound effect on certain aspects of its behaviour. The three main processes of cancer (growth, invasion and metastasis) have their equivalents in normal tissues. Most cancers are diagnosed by virtue of their morphological similarity to the tissue of origin. At the genetic level, with the exception of deletions, all necessary information is preserved, and the defective portion of DNA is relatively small. The key processes of malignancy are genetically controlled by the under or over expression of normal genes and their products that normally serve essential cellular functions such as the response to wounding. In addition, pathological and autopsy studies have suggested that most of the occult tumours in breast (and prostate cancers) may never reach clinical significance. A continuous growth model of breast cancer fails to explain the clinical data. The new model is based on the concept of tumour dormancy/latency both in the preclinical phase within the breast and later with the metastases that seed in the early phase of the natural history of the disease, once the primary focus has developed its microvasculature. The latter remain dormant until some signal – perhaps the act of surgery or other adverse life-event stimulates them into fast growth. Groups of cells without the potential to stimulate their own blood vessel supply can grow but remain small (up to 10^5 or 10^6 cells). The metastatic focus may grow quickly if (i) a subset of these cells switches on the signal for blood vessel growth (angiogenesis) and/or (ii) the natural inhibition of angiogenesis is removed. The model suggests that the metastatic development of unperturbed breast cancer is a sequential evolution from a non-angiogenic to an angiogenic state, with random transitions from one state to the next.

This model may explain the early peak of hazard function for local and distant recurrences in patients whose tumours are resected by combining the natural metastatic development of unperturbed disease ("the Fisher effect") with the angiogenic signal following surgery (*"the Folkman effect"*)[**]. It also correlates well with the findings of a modest benefit after adjuvant systemic chemotherapy.

We can now add a new mathematical model to the biological model described above. Breast cancer is like a complex organism existing in a state of dynamic equilibrium within the host, the equilibrium being very precarious and close to a chaotic boundary. Furthermore, the mathematics to describe the natural history of these "organisms" invokes nonlinear dynamics or chaos theory. This model is the first attempt to apply the new mathematics of complexity to make predictions about the factors influencing the natural history of breast cancer, which might one day provide a therapeutic window.

Central to the understanding of this model is the pioneering work of Folkman on tumour angiogenesis. As we know, solid tumours cannot grow beyond 10^6 cells or about 1–2 mm in diameter in the absence of a blood supply. The initial pre-vascular phase of growth is followed by a vascular phase in which tumour-induced angiogenesis is the rate-limiting step for further growth and provides malignant cells direct access to the circulation. In addition to the importance of the microvasculature, we can also visualize these microscopic foci as existing in a 'soup' of cytokines (biological molecules that signal or trigger cellular responses), with cells interacting with each other and with the surrounding stroma, interpreting competing signals directing the cancer cells in the direction of proliferation or apoptosis. Such complexity cannot be modelled by linear dynamics, or even a full understanding of the complete catalogue of genetic mutations at the cellular level, because the critical events of multiple cell-to-cell interactions require a thorough understanding of epigenetic phenomena.

What we now have is a new model of the disease that owes its genesis in part to the interpretation of the results of natural history

---

[**]*We chose to honour the late Judah Folkman from Harvard University in this way as he was responsible for most of the early basic research governing the mechanisms of angiogenesis. He deserved a Nobel prize for these discoveries.*

databases or clinical trials by way of hazard rate plots rather than life table curves. We can now see a new signal appearing against background noise that challenges the assumption of linear dynamics in favour of non-linear mathematics or chaos theory. This "signal" is the early peak of hazard for relapse that follows surgery within 48 months, whereas the near constant hazard thereafter might be the "echo" of the natural history of breast cancer left unperturbed by surgical interference.

If that is true then the act of wounding the patient creates a favourable environment for the sudden transfer of a metastasis from a latent to an active phase.

I now believe that careful reconsideration of both the therapeutic and deleterious effects of the wounding associated with breast cancer resection is required. Breast cancer and the women who bear it comprise a complex system. The dynamics of the system are not linear. The entry into this complex system by any potentially therapeutic intervention could have very different outcomes depending upon the conditions of the complex dynamic host-cancer relationship at the time of the intervention.

The therapeutic consequences of the new models are almost self-evident. The intervention that suggests itself would be anti-angiogenic, and the timing of the intervention would be preoperative, so that at the time of surgery the system is primed to protect against sudden flooding with angiogenic signals. (Indeed, some of the success attributed to adjuvant tamoxifen, arimidex or chemotherapy might be a result of their anti-angiogenic potential rather than cytostatic/ cytocidal effects.

Assuming we can protect the subject from the first peak of metastatic outgrowth, we will then have to monitor her with extreme vigilance. By the time the metastases are clinically apparent it is perhaps too late, therefore monitoring the patient with tumour markers and reintroducing an anti-angiogenic strategy at the first rise might prove successful. In the meantime we can continue to add additional layers of complexity to the simulations of our mathematical model in order to help develop alternative strategies for biological interventions to maintain the disease in equilibrium until nature takes its cull in old age.

****

I became a fellow of the Royal College of Surgeons in 1965 and retired from clinical practice in 2008. I started my career treating breast cancer with a Halsted radical mastectomy and now end my career by beginning to question whether surgery has any role in the cure of the disease. Along the way I have contributed to the knowledge base that raised the importance of medical and radiological treatment above my own noble discipline. Rather than becoming a pariah it seems that my life's work has been appreciated. In 2007 I was awarded the St Gallen prize, the most prestigious award in breast cancer research in the world. The little university town of St Gallen in eastern Switzerland plays host every two years to the most important breast cancer conference in Europe. It always takes place in the ski season and attracts the top researchers from all over the world for, in addition to improving their knowledge of oncology, they can also improve their skills in staying upright on a pair of planks pointing down a mountainside. The prize consisted of a large cheque (Figure 60), a beautiful Rolex watch, and of course the heady honour of following in the footsteps of my heroes, Bernie Fisher, Gianni Bonadonna and Umberto Veronesi. As I made my acceptance speech to an audience of 5,000, I thanked all the women in my life. My

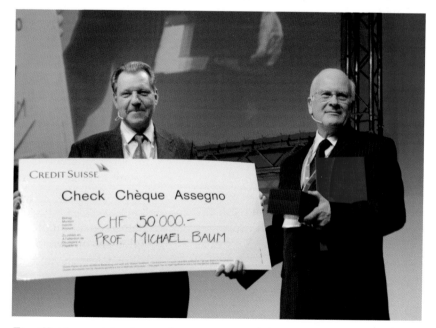

Fig. 60 Me receiving large cheque as part of the St Gallen prize

mother and my sister who galvanized my activity, my wife looking radiantly beautiful in the front row for supporting me through thick and thin, my loyal secretary Ciara McNulty who acted as my PA and guard dog for the last 20 years, and Mrs Hazel Thornton, a leading consumer advocate who has always actively supported my heretical views. Mrs Thornton is a Miss Marples-like character, those colleagues who try to patronize her should be careful, be *very* careful. Finally I thanked the unsung heroes of this story, the thousands of women with breast cancer who selflessly volunteered for the clinical trials for the sake of future generations and without whom I couldn't have completed my odyssey.

As for the large cheque, I blew it on a Chagall print and a huge 70th birthday party for all my friends and family.

Chapter 20

The Meaning of Life and other Easy Questions

"Tomorrow and tomorrow and tomorrow creeps in this petty pace from day to day to the last syllable of recorded time and all our yesterdays have lighted fools the way to dusty death. Out, out brief candle! Life's but a walking shadow. A poor player that struts and frets his hour upon the stage until he is heard no more. It is a tale told by an idiot full of sound and fury signifying nothing."

Macbeth Act V Scene V.

I learnt this soliloquy from Macbeth by heart at about the age of seven and used it as my "party piece" whenever my parents had the opportunity to show off their gifted children in front of an appreciative audience of family and friends. What my parents could never have predicted was the consequence of my sudden understanding of this bleak passage; when, at about the age of eleven, I embarked on my lifelong career as an insomniac. I remember clearly as a precocious young boy, lying awake all night trying to determine which was worse, to live forever, or to die at some uncertain point in the future, and what was life all about anyway? Shakespeare's suggestion that it signified nothing added a new layer or terror to my troubled nights. However, with the passage of time and my experience of life (and for that matter my experience of death), I think I've been able to define the questions with considerably more maturity than that of the pre-pubescent lad. I therefore welcomed the opportunity this memoir provides me with, to try to synthesize fifty years of self-questioning as to the meaning of life and the relevance of this to my clinical practice.

My attitude to the big question has been shaped by three major influences. These influences have been my upbringing as a Jew, my scientific curiosity as a practising clinical scientist, and my lifelong passionate affair with the visual arts. I don't think it's any exaggeration or particular conceit to say that sometimes I have to draw on all these inner resources in counselling my patients to help them make difficult decisions that might influence both the length and quality of their lives.

In the quiet doldrums between Christmas and the end of the New Year holiday break in 1995 I was summoned urgently to the Royal Free Hospital by my friend and colleague Dr. Alison Jones, to help a young woman make one of the toughest choices that anyone can ever be called upon to decide. In fact the decision reminded me of "Sophie's Choice" in William Styron's tragic novel of the same name.

The young woman in question was a pretty Greek Orthodox woman aged thirty-one. Four years earlier she had been diagnosed with breast cancer at a time when she was twelve weeks pregnant. The pregnancy was terminated and she underwent a conventional course of treatment that involved surgery, radiotherapy and chemotherapy. She was very keen to start a family and I advised her to wait a year or two. (It should be noted in passing that a pregnancy after breast cancer has been treated does not influence the prognosis, contrary to popular myth.) At the time I was called in to advise, she was twenty-one weeks pregnant and had already felt the quickening of the baby in her womb. Tragically, she had also felt the symptoms of the secondary cancer in her spine. In addition to the severe pain that she experienced, she also described numbness and paresis affecting her left arm. Investigations demonstrated that there were metastases in the spine, compressing the spinal cord and the nerve roots to her left arm. The various therapeutic options we had to consider included surgery for immediate decompression of the spinal cord, radiotherapy to the vertebra and cytotoxic chemotherapy. To do nothing at that stage would have been unthinkable as without treatment she would have become paraplegic in about 48 hours. Yet the most effective treatments to prevent this dreaded complication and to add to the length and quality to her remaining life would compromise the health or viability of the baby in the womb. Whose life was of greater value and whose decision was it anyway? Was the potential life of the unborn more meaningful than prolonging the life of a young adult? I was hoping that her own religious beliefs would guide me in this tough decision, but when asked directly she confessed to being a lapsed Christian and asked me for all the facts so that she could make an informed choice. Amongst the difficult truths that I had to convey was the fact that with even the best of all treatments her expectation of life would be unlikely to exceed two years and therefore should she allow a new life into the world the baby would grow up motherless. There was clearly no correct answer to this dilemma and I will return to the conclusion of this sad story at the end of the book but first let me tell what influenced my advice.

Judaic Influences

All we know for sure is this life and the history of other lives. Life after death is purely speculative and Jews do not believe that this life is a preparation for the afterlife. Yet in spite of that, there is an almost unspoken assumption amongst Jews that they will be rewarded for a virtuous life, after death. For example, the prayer in the house of mourning: *"Have mercy upon him. Pardon all his transgressions for there is none righteous upon the earth who doeth only good and sinneth not. Remember unto him the righteousness that he wrought and let his reward be with him and his recompense before him – bestow upon him the abounding happiness that is treasured up for the righteous"*. And yet paradoxically, on leaving the house of mourning our greeting to the principal mourners is to wish them a long life. We believe that life is of infinite worth and as infinity cannot be split then every moment of a life is of infinite value. We are therefore commanded to strive to preserve and prolong life and to avoid hazardous activities that risk our lives (and that should include smoking). This also explains our contempt for the suicide bombers, those who send them on their way and those who worship them as martyrs.

There are of course some mystical Chasidic sects who wish to explore the meaning of life and speculate on the afterlife, but mainstream Judaism accepts life as an end in itself and our religious teachings are primarily aimed at providing a code of conduct with more attention being paid to the relationships between man and man than between man and his God. Even to question whether life has a meaning may be a meaningless question to a Jew. If life is an end in itself then to question its meaning is as empty an exercise as to question the meaning of virtue, truth and beauty. If there is a meaning to life then it has to be beyond our comprehension however many subtle clues may pass across our consciousness. We are analogous to the fish trying to comprehend life on earth when all its fish-like brain can perceive are distorted two-dimensional images that appear in its firmament. I would even go further and suggest it is the ultimate in intellectual arrogance to "know" the answer to this question. I happen to note that there is a tendency amongst those who "know" with certainty to impose their beliefs on others and this in my opinion is the source of most of the world's problems. This confident knowledge of the unknowable leads to religious fundamentalism, forced conversion, terrorism and the three horsemen of the apocalypse.

The Teachings of Biological Science

It is natural for human beings to see patterns in their life. For every effect they like to know the cause. For example, is cancer a punishment? Is it a fault of lifestyle? Is it in the family? Why me? For every patient therefore, there is an emotional need to understand a little about the nature of cancer, if only to remove the guilt and the stigma, which has been associated with it in the past. The etiology of cancer probably involves two basic steps: *initiation,* which may be a necessary but not sufficient cause, and a second set of events, which are described as *promotional.* Apart from the rare cases of genetic predisposition to cancer, initiating factors are exogenous (from without) whereas promotional factors are largely constitutional (from within). There are some obvious examples where clearly defined exogenous factors initiate the disease and where in theory prevention is possible. The best example of course is smoking and its impact on the incidence of lung cancer, bladder cancer and head and neck cancer. Another well established example of this kind is the association between malignant melanoma of the skin and the exposure of white races to excessive sunlight. It is likely that the initiation of the majority of common and, for that matter, uncommon cancers, are random events resulting from exogenous factors beyond our control leading to somatic mutations in the human genome. These may result from cosmic rays, radon from the granite of the earth or the low, persistent background of x-radiation. We assume that there are constant random mutations occurring within our genome, but we have exquisite repair mechanisms and to an extent our vulnerability to cancer may not be so much due to the exogenous factors as to inherent failures of our natural repair mechanisms. We are thus rapidly developing a mechanistic concept of the nature of cancer, which will ultimately lead to rational biological cures. In the meantime, we have to ask whether this increasing knowledge can help us understand cancer from the humanistic point of view. How can a cancer doctor retain any semblance of faith, which is tested each time he witnesses the suffering imposed by this dreadful disease. Paradoxically, each time I contemplate the micro-cosmos of the cancer cell, I find my faith restored. Of course it is commonplace to see God's work in the cosmos as illustrated by the last paragraph of Stephen Hawking's best seller "A Brief History of Time": *"There may be only one complete unified theory that is self-consistent and allows the existence of structures as complicated as human beings who can investigate the laws of the universe and ask about the nature of God. If we find the answer to that, it would be the ultimate triumph of human reason, for then we would know the mind of God"*. As described already, I enjoy the same sense of awe from the study of inner space rather than outer space. Watson and Crick discovered the structure of DNA in 1953 and subsequent biological scientists have come up with mind-boggling statistics as awe inspiring as those related to cosmology. Richard Dawkins puts it this way.... there are 3×10^{12} cells in the body and 46 chromosomes per cell. 2 metres of DNA are packed into the nucleus of each cell tightly wound on these chromosomes. That is 6×10^{12} meters of DNA in each body, which is equivalent to the distance to the moon and back 8000 times! Each time the cell divides there is the hazard of a somatic mutation as a random event. Some cells divide every 48 hours. It is therefore a miracle to me that life can be sustained at all and the question "why me?" whenever someone develops cancer should be turned on its head and every day of everyone's life we should offer up a prayer that we *didn't* develop cancer in the previous 24 hours. Richard Dawkins in his most readable and mischievous book "The Blind Watchmaker" describes the fidelity of the transcription process beautifully and I wish to quote one of his passages at length: *"DNA's performance as an archival medium is spectacular. In its capacity to preserve a message it far outdoes tablets of stone. Letters carved on gravestones become unreadable in mere hundreds of years. The DNA document is even more impressive, because unlike tablets of stone it is not the same physical structure that lasts and preserves the text. It is repeatedly being copied and recopied as the generations go by, like the Hebrew*

Scriptures, which were ritually copied by scribes every eighty years to forestall their wearing out. It is hard to estimate how many times the DNA document has been recopied in our lineage; probably as many as twenty billion times. It is hard to find a yardstick with which to compare the preservation of more than 99% of the information in twenty billion successive copyings."

Such precision is miraculous. Life in the first place is miraculous and preservation of our species is miraculous. Cancer is the inevitable result of any instability within the human genome without which evolution would have been postponed. Cancer therefore is the inevitable result of the gift of life and the evolution of a species to its current state of self-awareness that allows it to ask such questions. We should therefore give thanks for this gift however brief the candle within our grasp. It is of course a mute point as to whom or what we give thanks. That is another question mischievously addressed by Richard Dawkins, in his book "The God Delusion". That aside one could therefore say that in asking the question "What is the meaning of life?" we are effectively looking a gift horse in the mouth. It could then be argued why have I been wasting my time as a clinical scientist?

I have given you the biologist's reason to believe, which includes a belief in reason but I also believe in something transcendental (*pace Dawkins*) which encourages me to challenge nature.

Lessons from the Study of Fine Art

If life is a miracle, a gift and an end in itself, how do we judge a good life and for how long should we try to extend that life? It is to address these fundamental questions that I have to turn to the arts for guidance. Great works of art, whether they are paintings, music or literature, are judged by their capacity to illustrate, interpret and enhance life's experience. I would like to take this definition and use fine art itself as the metaphor to set the parameters for a good and appropriately lengthy life. When judging a great painting I look for harmony of composition, balance of colour and tone and its capacity to evoke emotions of joy or understanding, but even someone unschooled in the appreciation of fine art can recognize an unfinished work when he sees it. For example, Leonardo da Vinci's Adoration of the King's in the Uffizi Gallery, Florence: this has perfect composition and perspective and certain areas are beautifully sketched in, namely the heads of the Magi and some rearing horses in the distance, yet it is clearly unfinished. Apart from areas of ground colour there is little else to give it depth or please the eye with harmony of hue. One despairs that so many of Leonardo's works remained unfinished, yet all are tributes to his flawed genius.

I believe life should be worked upon as with any other expression of the human craving to produce perfection. A good life can be judged at any one time by its horizontal harmonies judged by relationships with family and friends, satisfaction with work or professional advancement and the capacity to enjoy leisure and recreation. Looking at life vertically a complete and balanced composition would include a time for childhood games, a time for education, a time for marriage and homebuilding, a time for the conception and raising of children, a time to hand over to the next generation, to retire and enjoy the fruits of one's labour and finally a time for a dignified death. Not all of us are capable of creating great works of art, but there is an art in the striving for achievement and even a tragically foreshortened life can leave beauty behind like an unfinished symphony.

My brother David (Figure 61)

Let me remind you about my young brother David. He had a lean and hungry look crowned by a huge head of curly hair that made one think of Harpo Marx. He wore exuberant bow ties, did magic and was a deeply religious Jew, indeed a *"Shomer Shabbat"*. (Literally meaning Guardian of the Sabbath). In contrast I am portly and balding, I wear normal ties and respect those laws of the Sabbath that suit me. We came from the same genetic pool but were of different phenotypes and yet in parts our brains seemed to have been hard-wired in a similar way. He was also a clinical scientist but a pediatrician. He was a fanatically hard worker and set the pace when we used to study together as undergraduates and young post grads in Birmingham. He went on to great things and died as President of the Royal College of Pediatrics and Child Health.

On his death he left behind him his wife Angela, an artist, and four wonderful boys, Benjamin (Buzz), Joshua, Jacob and Samuel. It was only at his memorial service in Bristol, attended by thousands, that I learnt of all his achievements in promoting children's health around the globe and the promotion of the hospice movement for children dying of cancer. He combined a zeal for life fuelled by his faith and his candle burnt out prematurely flaming at both ends. But *what a life*, a masterpiece of a life, a life full of colour and perfect symmetry yet in many ways an unfinished symphony of a life. He

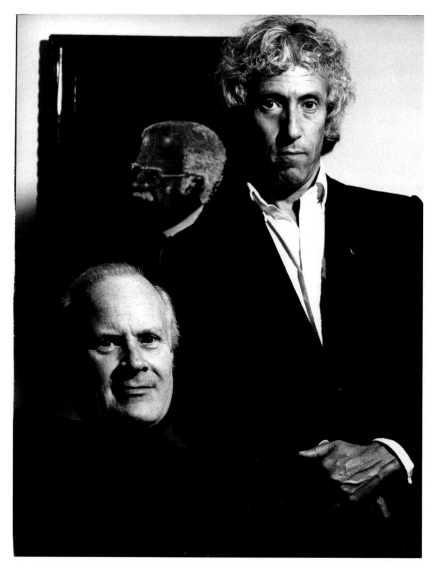

Fig. 61 My brother David and I, From the Sunday Times

never lived to enjoy that golden retirement he dreamed of, with him studying Talmud in S'fad in Northern Galilee with Angela painting by his side. The nearest he came to that was his burial plot in Rosh Pinah overlooking his beloved Kineret (The Sea of Galilee). Yet in his foreshortened life he achieved more than most could achieve if they lived to be 120.

The Rajasthani Potter

In October 1994 my wife and I visited India to take in the UICC World Cancer Congress in New Delhi. We took advantage of this visit to enjoy a very comfortable and spectacular tour of the Golden Triangle in Rajasthan. On this visit I learnt that of the population of India, which numbers well over one billion, seven hundred and fifty million live in abject poverty with a life expectancy thirty years less than our own. One cannot possibly begin to imagine the enormity of such numbers and once again it is necessary in order to gain the slightest of insights, to focus in on the life of a single individual. We enjoyed three magnificent days staying in the lap of luxury in the Lake Palace Hotel in Udaipur. On one of these days our guide took us through the hills and jungle north of Udaipur to visit the Jain Temples of Ranakpur. Along the way he made a diversion so that we could visit a small rural village where he was well known. Stopping at the side of a rutted and primitive road we continued our journey on foot through all kinds of excreta and rubbish past stagnant pools where the colourful women of Rajasthan were beating their saris clean; through a tumbledown village of mud-bricks and collapsing thatch to a little shed to watch the potter at his work. As always, I enjoyed the creation of an artifact out of formless clay. The potter enjoyed our interest and his wife and countless children were thrilled by the visit of alien creatures from what might have been another planet. Their interest and amusement with us and the offers of hospitality were disarmingly genuine. This seemed to be a man, happy with the weft of his life strengthened by his family network and the beauty and utility of the objects he was creating. Also, from what I learned during my visit to India, the warp of his life was punctuated by Hindu festivals and rituals. Like many of the poor and uneducated in India, he was blissfully unaware of the alternative lifestyle enjoyed by us Westerners and so probably lacked the ambition to "improve himself" and had no desire for consumer durables or skiing holidays. I am well aware that it is easy to romanticize this squalor and look upon this harmless man as a "noble savage", but just as we should try and improve on nature with finding a cure for cancer I believe it should be an expression of our humanity to improve upon nurture so that the health and welfare of this family could be improved. I cannot believe that his life would lose much of value if all his children had a good education and were able to realize their full potential and enjoy the artistic traditions of their own society. I don't believe anything of value would be lost by trying to reduce the appalling infant mortality by the simple expedient of providing fresh, uncontaminated running water, and I cannot believe that much of value would be lost if the potter lived long enough to enjoy his grandchildren. This then leaves me with a troubling thought. Would India, or for that matter, the rest of the world, be a better place if there were fewer citizens with more complete lives. In other words is birth control and easy access to abortion the only answers to these questions. I certainly don't side with the pro-life fanatics in the United States of America. I can think of no greater obscenity than those who commit murder in the name of the unborn. I tend to side with the sardonic political commentator P J O'Rourke. In his book "All the World's Troubles" he points out with devastating logic that population density per se is not the cause of poverty and misery and emphasizes that certain areas of southern California have a greater population density than the Delta area of Bangladesh. His explanation for the cause of poverty, misery and a high infant mortality is the direct correlation of these world troubles with nations that practice religious intolerance, feudalism and corruption.

Returning now to my metaphor of the weft and warp of life; I recognise that to describe life as a rich tapestry is a rather exhausted cliché, but it will serve my purpose now. A character in Somerset Maugham's lovely novel, loosely based on the life of Gauguin, "The Moon and Sixpence", carries with him at all times a rolled up Persian carpet. He uses this as a "memento vitae". It had always been my ambition to emulate this character and one of the other great successes of our visit to India was to bring back a silken Kashmiri carpet. Due to some brilliant bargaining on behalf of my wife we were able to purchase this exquisite work of art at barely twice what it cost the vendor! Like all true Kashmiri silk carpets it is indeed magic. Viewed from my current position at my writing desk I can enjoy its robust and intricate patterns suggestive of the mathematics of a complex organism. The colours are vivid, rich and dark. Viewed from the other side, it takes on an entirely different character. The shades are pastel, the outlines of the design ephemeral and the carpet appears to float above the ground. Give me my current perspective of this carpet any day and let the metaphysicians enjoy the alternative viewpoint as much as they like, providing they don't impose their view of life on me by forced conversion, torture or decree.

Returning to the Case in Point

Let me now return to the case of the young woman twenty one weeks' pregnant with impending spinal cord compression from metastatic breast cancer. As an informed and carefully calculated choice she allowed the pregnancy to go to thirty two weeks before delivery through Caesarean section. This compromise allowed a new life into the world with an almost 100% chance of survival in health to adult life. This child is a reminder to her husband of his late wife. This child allows a beautiful symmetry in her foreshortened life denied on the previous occasion at the time of her initial diagnosis. I supported her in this decision from my own ethical standpoint because I was not actively shortening her life for the benefit of the child. This new life started at a disadvantage because of the limited life expectancy of the mother, but the starting point for all works of art are of an infinite variety and what could be a less promising subject than say Van Gogh's shoes? Although as a Jew I will always value the life of a mother over the potential life of a foetus, I can recognize the persuasiveness of the argument that a potential life may be valued equally with the fully developed life of the adult.

****

Twenty-five years ago I suffered a severe bout of clinical depression. Only fellow sufferers will fully appreciate what this mean. That mood is certainly well illustrated in the passage from Macbeth quoted at the start of this chapter. No amount of reassurance from my family or friends could persuade me that I was of any worth and that my life had any meaning. Although frightful at that time I think that period of illness was of enormous and lasting value to me. Many people live their life taking it for granted without truly valuing the gift. There is no better way of describing my attitude to life than by using the words of George Bernard Shaw whose feelings are the complete antithesis to those Shakespeare expressed through the mouth of Macbeth:

"This is the true joy in life, the being used for a purpose recognized by yourself as a mighty one, the being a force of nature instead of a feverish little clod of ailments and grievances complaining that the world will not devote itself to making you happy. I am of the opinion that my life belongs to the whole community, and as long as I live it is my privilege to do for it whatever I can. I want to be thoroughly used up when I die, for the harder I work the more I live. I rejoice in life for its own sake. Life is no brief candle to me. It is a sort of splendid torch which I have got hold of for the moment and I want to make it burn as brightly as possible before handing it on to future generations."

That was how my brother David lived his life and thus was the manner of his parting.

Index